Jerry D. Marx (Ed.)

Reinventing Healthy Communities: Implications for Individual and Societal Well-Being

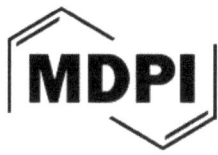

This book is a reprint of the Special Issue that appeared in the online, open access journal, *Social Sciences* (ISSN 2076-0760) from 2015–2016, available at:

http://www.mdpi.com/journal/socsci/special_issues/reinventing_realthy_communities

Guest Editor
Jerry D. Marx
Department of Social Work, University of New Hampshire
USA

Editorial Office
MDPI AG
St. Alban-Anlage 66
Basel, Switzerland

Publisher
Shu-Kun Lin

Assistant Editor
Siyang Liu

1. Edition 2016

MDPI • Basel • Beijing • Wuhan • Barcelona • Belgrade

ISBN 978-3-03842-262-4 (Hbk)
ISBN 978-3-03842-263-1 (PDF)

Articles in this volume are Open Access and distributed under the Creative Commons Attribution license (CC BY), which allows users to download, copy and build upon published articles even for commercial purposes, as long as the author and publisher are properly credited, which ensures maximum dissemination and a wider impact of our publications. The book taken as a whole is © 2016 MDPI, Basel, Switzerland, distributed under the terms and conditions of the Creative Commons by Attribution (CC BY-NC-ND) license (http://creativecommons.org/licenses/by-nc-nd/4.0/).

Table of Contents

List of Contributors V

About the Guest Editor IX

Jerry D. Marx
Healthy Communities: What Have We Learned and Where do We Go from Here?
Reprinted from: *Soc. Sci.* **2016**, *5*(3), 44
http://www.mdpi.com/2076-0760/5/3/44 1

Mark Roseland and Maria Spiliotopoulou
Converging Urban Agendas: Toward Healthy and Sustainable Communities
Reprinted from: *Soc. Sci.* **2016**, *5*(3), 28
http://www.mdpi.com/2076-0760/5/3/28 6

Jerry Marx and Alison Rataj
A Case Study in Organizing for Livable and Sustainable Communities
Reprinted from: *Soc. Sci.* **2016**, *5*(1), 1
http://www.mdpi.com/2076-0760/5/1/1 35

Rachel Robinson
Hybridity: A Theory of Agency in Early Childhood Governance
Reprinted from: *Soc. Sci.* **2016**, *5*(1), 9
http://www.mdpi.com/2076-0760/5/1/9 45

Mary Moeller, Angela McKillip, Ruth Wienk and Kay Cutler
In Pursuit of Child and Family Well-Being: Initial Steps to Advocacy
Reprinted from: *Soc. Sci.* **2016**, *5*(3), 30
http://www.mdpi.com/2076-0760/5/3/30 63

Kisha Holden, Tabia Akintobi, Jammie Hopkins, Allyson Belton, Brian McGregor, Starla Blanks and Glenda Wrenn
Community Engaged Leadership to Advance Health Equity and Build Healthier Communities
Reprinted from: *Soc. Sci.* **2016**, 5(1), 2
http://www.mdpi.com/2076-0760/5/1/2 80

Kristy Buccieri
Integrated Social Housing and Health Care for Homeless and Marginally-Housed Individuals: A Study of the Housing and Homelessness Steering Committee in Ontario, Canada
Reprinted from: *Soc. Sci.* **2016**, 5(2), 15
http://www.mdpi.com/2076-0760/5/2/15 105

Vernon B. Carter and Jerry D. Marx
U.S. Volunteering in the Aftermath of the Great Recession: Were African Americans a Significant Factor?
Reprinted from: *Soc. Sci.* **2016**, 5(2), 22
http://www.mdpi.com/2076-0760/5/2/22 129

Isabelle Laurin, Angèle Bilodeau, Nadia Giguère and Louise Potvin
Intersectoral Mobilization in Child Development: An Outcome Assessment of the Survey of the School Readiness of Montreal Children
Reprinted from: *Soc. Sci.* **2015**, 4(4), 1316–1334
http://www.mdpi.com/2076-0760/4/4/1316 150

Ahmed Shoukry Rashad and Mesbah Fathy Sharaf
Who Benefits from Public Healthcare Subsidies in Egypt?
Reprinted from: *Soc. Sci.* **2015**, 4(4), 1162–1176
http://www.mdpi.com/2076-0760/4/4/1162 172

Hazel Williams-Roberts, Bonnie Jeffery, Shanthi Johnson and Nazeem Muhajarine
The Effectiveness of Healthy Community Approaches on Positive Health Outcomes in Canada and the United States
Reprinted from: *Soc. Sci.* **2016**, 5(1), 3
http://www.mdpi.com/2076-0760/5/1/3 190

List of Contributors

Tabia Akintobi Prevention Research Center, and Department of Community Health and Preventive Medicine, Morehouse School of Medicine, 720 Westview Drive, Atlanta, GA 30310, USA.

Allyson Belton Satcher Health Leadership Institute, Morehouse School of Medicine, 720 Westview Drive, Atlanta, GA 30310, USA.

Angèle Bilodeau School of Public Health, University of Montreal, PO Box 6128 Station Centre-ville, Montreal, QC H3C 3J7, Canada.

Starla Blanks Satcher Health Leadership Institute, Morehouse School of Medicine, 720 Westview Drive, Atlanta, GA 30310, USA.

Kristy Buccieri Department of Sociology, Trent University, 1600 W Bank Dr, Peterborough, ON K9J 0G2, Canada.

Vernon B. Carter Department of Social Work, University of New Hampshire, Durham, NH 03824, USA.

Kay Cutler Department of Teaching, Learning & Leadership, South Dakota State University, Brookings, SD 57007, USA.

Nadia Giguère Jeanne-Mance Health and Social Services Center Research Center, 1250 Sanguinet Street, Suite 477, Montreal, QC H2X 3E7, Canada.

Kisha Holden Department of Community Health and Preventive Medicine, Satcher Health Leadership Institute, and Department of Psychiatry & Behavioral Science, Morehouse School of Medicine, 720 Westview Drive, Atlanta, GA 30310, USA.

Jammie Hopkins Department of Community Health and Preventive Medicine, and Satcher Health Leadership Institute, Morehouse School of Medicine, 720 Westview Drive, Atlanta, GA 30310, USA.

Bonnie Jeffery Faculty of Social Work, Saskatchewan Population Health and Evaluation Research Unit, University of Regina, Prince Albert Campus, Saskatchewan S6V 7S3, Canada.

Shanthi Johnson Faculty of Kinesiology and Health Studies, Saskatchewan Population Health and Evaluation Research Unit, University of Regina, Regina, Saskatchewan S4S 0A2, Canada.

Isabelle Laurin Montreal Department of Public Health, 1301 Sherbrooke East, Montreal, QC H2L 1M3, Canada.

Jerry D. Marx Department of Social Work, University of New Hampshire, Hood House, 89 Main St., Durham, NH 03824, USA.

Brian McGregor Satcher Health Leadership Institute, and Department of Psychiatry & Behavioral Science, Morehouse School of Medicine, 720 Westview Drive, Atlanta, GA 30310, USA.

Angela McKillip School of Design, South Dakota State University, Brookings, SD 57007, USA.

Mary Moeller Department of Teaching, Learning & Leadership, South Dakota State University, Brookings, SD 57007, USA.

Nazeem Muhajarine Community Health and Epidemiology, Saskatchewan Population Health and Evaluation Research Unit, University of Saskatchewan, Saskatoon, Saskatchewan S7N 5E5, Canada.

Louise Potvin School of Public Health, University of Montreal, PO Box 6128 Station Centre-ville, Montreal, QC H3C 3J7, Canada.

Ahmed Shoukry Rashad Department of Economics, Faculty of Commerce, Damanhour University, Damanhour 22514, Egypt.

Alison Rataj Department of Social Work, University of New Hampshire, Durham, NH 03824, USA.

Rachel Robinson School of Social and Political Sciences, University of Melbourne, Melbourne, VIC 3000, Australia.

Mark Roseland Centre for Sustainable Community Development, School of Resource and Environmental Management, Simon Fraser University, Burnaby, BC V5A 1S6, Canada.

Mesbah Fathy Sharaf Department of Economics, Faculty of Arts, University of Alberta, Edmonton, AB T6G 2H4, Canada; Department of Economics, Faculty of Commerce, Damanhour University, Damanhour 22514, Egypt.

Maria Spiliotopoulou Centre for Sustainable Community Development, School of Resource and Environmental Management, Simon Fraser University, Burnaby, BC V5A 1S6, Canada.

Ruth Wienk Sociology Department, South Dakota State University, Brookings, SD 57007, USA.

Hazel Williams-Roberts Community Health and Epidemiology, University of Saskatchewan, Saskatoon, Saskatchewan S7N 5E5, Canada.

Glenda Wrenn Satcher Health Leadership Institute, and Department of Psychiatry & Behavioral Science, Morehouse School of Medicine, 720 Westview Drive, Atlanta, GA 30310, USA.

About the Guest Editor

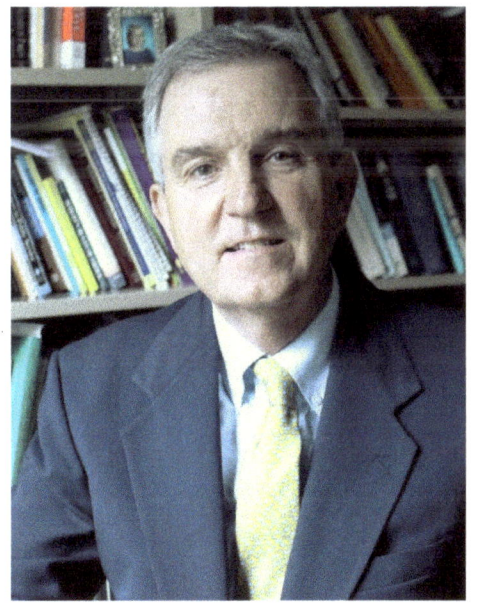

Jerry D. Marx, Ph.D., is a tenured, Associate Professor in the Department of Social Work at the University of New Hampshire (U.N.H.). He also currently serves as the Faculty Director of the University of New Hampshire Honors Program. Dr. Marx's research focuses on social policy and administration with an emphasis on community-based nonprofit organizations. He has published journal articles on such topics as human service volunteerism and the charitable giving patterns of corporations, women, African Americans, and Hispanic Americans. Marx's scholarship resulted in a college research award in 1999 and an invitation to the first White House Conference on Philanthropy in 1999. His textbooks are "Social Work and Social Welfare: An Introduction," co-authored by Anne Broussard, Fleur Hopper, and Dave Worster and published by Pearson (2011) as well as "Social Welfare: The American Partnership," published by Allyn & Bacon in 2004. Before earning his Ph.D., he served for eight years in executive leadership positions in the nonprofit sector.

Healthy Communities: What Have We Learned and Where do We Go from Here?

Jerry D. Marx

> Reprinted from *Soc. Sci.* Cite as: Marx, J.D. Healthy Communities: What Have We Learned and Where do We Go from Here? *Soc. Sci.* **2016**, *5*, 44.

Systems theory [1,2] suggests that healthy communities promote healthy individual development. That is, healthy systems take care of their component parts, and they do this, in part, by conducting positive exchanges with external systems. However, the thinking on what characterizes a "healthy" community continues to change over time. Social exchange theory [3] emphasizes the norms of reciprocity and the underlying relationships of trust that develop in healthy communities. Other authors stress the need for various forms of capital, not only economic and political, but also social, environmental, cultural, and spiritual [4,5].

Contemporary theory underlying the trend towards "New Urbanism" [6] has its roots in the writings of Jane Jacobs [7]. Jacobs, a U.S. citizen, challenged the prevailing notions of urban planning in the United States, claiming that urban renewal of the 1940s and 1950s had hurt the health of cities due to single use zoning that located residents, parks, business, government services, etc. in separate sections of the city. This tended to leave these areas unused for extended periods of each day, thus isolating various groups and uses. She further insisted that high rise towers and open plazas created wind swept areas with little appeal to pedestrians, who preferred denser neighborhoods with short blocks and buildings of moderate height.

Consequently, contemporary views of "livable communities" maintain that density and diversity are good for the health of cities. Healthy communities are more pedestrian-friendly and less automobile-centric. Mixed-use zoning keeps a flow of people through streets, neighborhoods, and districts, which is good for business, safety, and tourism. Locally-sourced food is more sustainable for the environment and healthier for individuals [7–9].

But how does this all relate to the current and future provision of social services? And how should social institutions collaborate with those of the economic and political sectors to maximize individual and societal well-being? Those involved with the settlement house movement of the late 1800s and early 1900s in Great Britain and the United States certainly understood the impact of the environment on individual functioning and worked with both government and business leaders to better organize communities and services to meet the needs of residents. Deinstitutionalization and the movement toward community-based social services in the U.S. in the 1960s, 1970s, and 1980s recognized the potential positive influence of healthy communities on individual functioning [10,11].

This special collection, therefore, aims to focus on the contextual factors that characterize "healthy communities" and that impact individual development and well being around the world. Researchers from various fields including psychiatry, public health, sociology, political science, community planning, economics, kinesiology, and social work present their theoretical, empirical, or practice-based studies on critical issues involving healthy communities.

To begin, Roseland and Spiliotopoulou provide a historical overview of urban sustainability theory and practice, and explain why urban sustainability planning and development currently face limited and inconsistent application [12]. The authors argue that urban sustainability today needs "to embrace equity, inclusion, and other social considerations; encourage the integration of human and environmental health interests; and encompass triple-bottom-line-inspired outcomes." The authors, therefore, encourage a broad perspective on healthy communities that emphasizes social, financial as well as environmental goals.

Marx and Rataj in the second paper in this collection present a case study that illustrates this growing public concern for a broader paradigm in urban planning and community development [13]. The case study documents a successful community organizing effort to promote a more livable neighborhood in Portland, Maine (USA). In opposing a development project that had been endorsed by the city government, community activists stressed the importance of social and environmental factors impacting community health and livability. Implications for healthy communities, community activists, and social work educators are discussed.

Robinson provides a more theoretical paper on the topic of healthy communities [14]. That is, the author explores the relevance of "hybridity" for the "Kids in Communities" study—an Australian research project examining community influences on child development across multiple case study sites in that country.

Moeller, McKillip, Wienk, and Cutler also see children and families as central to sustaining healthy communities [15]. The authors provide a case study of one rural community in the U.S. that used an inquiry-based approach to address the question, "How can we engage our citizens to improve child and family well-being in our community?" Their paper describes the formation of a "community of practice," its growing links to community agencies, and its initial efforts to develop calls to action through participatory research and grassroots activism.

Holden et al. agree with Roseland and Spiliotopoulou that community health is a matter of equity and human rights [16]. They argue that addressing the complex health and well-being needs of ethnically and culturally diverse communities requires creative strategies to reduce risk factors and bolster protective factors. To this end, the authors examine strategic efforts to improve individual longevity and quality of life through accessible primary care, focused community-based programs, multi-disciplinary clinical and translational research, and effective health policy advocacy.

Buccieri contributes to this collection on reinventing healthy communities by providing a case study on planning for social housing and health care in Ontario, Canada [17]. Homelessness is a multi-dimensional social problem that requires a coordinated systems approach. In recent years, Canada has attempted to integrate health care and social care to better address the needs of homeless persons. This article documents the way in which planners for social housing and health care collaborated to align their system approaches for homeless persons.

The Great Recession created homelessness and other forms of hardship for vulnerable people in communities throughout the world. Although African Americans are generally especially hard hit by these types of economic crises, they have a long and distinctive history of community volunteerism and mutual assistance. Consequently, Carter and Marx examined African American volunteering in non-profit organizations in the aftermath of the 2008–2009 recession [18]. Specifically, the researchers use data from the Panel Study of Income Dynamics (PSID) to analyze U.S. volunteering in four categories of organizations: poverty organizations, senior service agencies, social action groups, and religious affiliated organizations. All of these organizations are part of social capital, and therefore, help to sustain healthy communities. The authors' secondary analysis produced significant findings regarding volunteerism among African Americans in these community-based organizations.

Like the Robinson study and the research by Moeller et al., Laurin, Bilodeau, Giguere, and Potvin address the topic of healthy communities from the perspective of child development. In this study, the researchers examined the decision-making process that fostered ownership of the results of the 2006 "Survey of the School Readiness of Montreal Children" [19]. Their analysis documents the impacts of those survey findings on intersectoral action regarding early childhood services. An important outcome has been closer collaboration between early childhood services and school systems. This includes the development of both transition-to-kindergarten tools and literacy activities. The authors discuss the implications for future community planning.

Rashad and Sharaf, like other authors in this collection, stress the importance of equity to the health of communities and society at large [20]. The findings of their quantitative study in Egypt reject the hypothesis that health care subsidies mostly benefit the poor. Consequently, the researchers conclude that future poverty reduction and healthcare reform efforts in Egypt should not only expand healthcare coverage, but also on improve the equity of its distribution for poor citizens.

In the final paper, Williams-Roberts, Jeffery, Johnson, and Muhajarine maintain that the concept of healthy communities actually involves a diverse set of strategies, making evaluation of health outcomes related to individual approaches critically important to sustaining such efforts [21]. Their systematic review analyzes the effectiveness in this regard of the ten most common healthy community approaches: Healthy Cities/Communities, Smart Growth, Child Friendly Cities, Safe Routes to Schools, Safe Communities, Active Living Communities, Livable Communities, Social Cities, Age-Friendly Cities, and Dementia Friendly Cities. Implications for future evaluative research are considered.

Conflicts of Interest: The author declares no conflict of interest.

References

1. Ludwig von Bertalanffy. *General Systems Theory: Foundations, Development, Applications*. New York: George Braziller, 1968.
2. Urie Bronfenbrenner. *The Ecology of Human Development: Experiments by Nature and Design*. Cambridge: Harvard University Press, 1979.
3. Peter M. Blau. *Exchange & Power in Social Life*. New York: Wiley, 1964.
4. Robert D. Putnam. *Bowling Alone: The Collapse and Revival of American Community*. New York: Simon and Schuster, 2000.
5. Mark Roseland. *Toward Sustainable Communities*. Gabriola Island: New Society, 2012.
6. New Urbanism. "Principles of Urbanism." Available online: http://www.newurbanism.org/newurbanism/principles.html (accessed on 24 August 2016).
7. Jane Jacobs. *The Death and Life of Great American Cities*. New York: Random House, 1961.
8. David Owen. *Green Metropolis: Why Living Smaller, Living Closer, and Driving Less are the Keys to Sustainability*. New York: Penguin Books, 2009.
9. Edward Glaeser. *Triumph of the City*. New York: Penguin, 2011.
10. Bruce Jansson. *The Reluctant Welfare State: Engaging History to Advance Social Work Practice in Contemporary Society*, 7th ed. Pacific Grove: Brooks Cole, 2011.
11. Jerry D. Marx. *Social Welfare: The American Partnership*. Boston: Allyn & Bacon, 2004.
12. Mark Roseland, and Maria Spiliotopoulou. "Converging Urban Agendas: Toward Healthy and Sustainable Communities." *Social Sciences* 5 (2016): 28.
13. Jerry D. Marx, and Alison Rataj. "A Case Study in Organizing for Livable and Sustainable Communities." *Social Sciences* 5 (2015): 1.
14. Rachel Robinson. "Hybridity: A Theory of Agency in Early Childhood Governance." *Social Sciences* 5 (2016): 9.
15. Mary Moeller, Angela McKillip, Ruth Wienk, and Kay Cutler. "In Pursuit of Child and Family Well-Being: Initial Steps to Advocacy." *Social Sciences* 5 (2016): 30.
16. Kisha Holden, Tabia Akintobi, Jammie Hopkins, Allyson Belton, Brian McGregor, Starla Blanks, and Glenda Wrenn. "Community Engaged Leadership to Advance Health Equity and Build Healthier Communities." *Social Sciences* 5 (2015): 2.

17. Kristy Buccieri. "Integrated Social Housing and Health Care for Homeless and Marginally-Housed Individuals: A Study of the Housing and Homelessness Steering Committee in Ontario, Canada." *Social Sciences* 5 (2016): 15.
18. Vernon B. Carter, and Jerry D. Marx. "US Volunteering in the Aftermath of the Great Recession: Were African Americans a Significant Factor? " *Social Sciences* 5 (2016): 22.
19. Isabelle Laurin, Angèle Bilodeau, Nadia Giguère, and Louise Potvin. "Intersectoral Mobilization in Child Development: An Outcome Assessment of the Survey of the School Readiness of Montreal Children." *Social Sciences* 4 (2015): 1316–34.
20. Ahmed Shoukry Rashad, and Mesbah Fathy Sharaf. "Who Benefits from Public Healthcare Subsidies in Egypt? " *Social Sciences* 4 (2015): 1162–76.
21. Hazel Williams-Roberts, Bonnie Jeffery, Shanthi Johnson, and Nazeem Muhajarine. "The Effectiveness of Healthy Community Approaches on Positive Health Outcomes in Canada and the United States." *Social Sciences* 5 (2015): 3.

Converging Urban Agendas: Toward Healthy and Sustainable Communities

Mark Roseland and Maria Spiliotopoulou

Abstract: In light of recent developments such as the COP21 Paris climate agreement, the UN adoption of the Sustainable Development Goals for 2030, and the Habitat III Conference, there is increasing recognition of the role of human settlements as key components of both global challenges and global solutions. "Urban sustainability" under various names has matured over the last three decades not only in planning and related fields, but also in wider professional and popular discourse. In this paper we trace a historical overview of urban sustainability theory and practice, and explain why urban sustainability planning and development currently face limited and inconsistent application. We show that this lack of public uptake is due in part to monitoring, assessment, and decision-support frameworks and tools that do not engage citizens and their governments in a shared "strong sustainability" analysis and/or vision. We argue that urban sustainability today clearly needs to embrace equity, inclusion, and other social considerations; contribute to constructive societal mobilisation and compelling policy-making; advocate for development as a better alternative to growth; encourage the integration of human and environmental health interests; and encompass triple-bottom-line-inspired outcomes. Focusing on community capital productivity and regeneration may be the key to advancing healthy and sustainable communities.

Reprinted from *Soc. Sci.* Cite as: Roseland, M.; Spiliotopoulou, M. Converging Urban Agendas: Toward Healthy and Sustainable Communities. *Soc. Sci.* **2016**, 5, 28.

1. Introduction

A growing number of scholars are referring to the modern period as "the Anthropocene", the era when human development is unfolding at a pace that is detrimental for our host planet [1]. A multitude of signs clearly indicate that the Earth cannot sustain the ever-growing human population; these signs include climate change and increased frequency of extreme phenomena; persistent poverty and inaccessibility to basic provisions like clean water and sanitation; and degradation of ecosystem services and species extinction at an unprecedented rate [2].

The argument that there should be limits to growth was established decades ago in the seminal report submitted by Meadows et al. to the Club of Rome [3], and it is finally gaining momentum [4,5]. We no longer live in an "empty world", but rather in a "full" one [6], with significant implications and repercussions for current and future generations. Current generations now have both the knowledge and the responsibility to lead humanity toward a more sustainable future [2].

In some cases the situation may not be irreversible; however, we now have more understanding of where the planetary boundaries are and, although some suggested thresholds seem to have been exceeded (genetic diversity, climate change, nitrogen cycle, and land-system change) [7], we need to make concerted efforts to remain within these interconnected boundaries [8]. According to current knowledge the Holocene is the only state of the Earth that can support human societies as we know them; human activity however has been extending the Earth's boundaries to the point that the planet as a system may lose it resilience, i.e., it may not be able to sustain the increasing anthropogenic pressure [7].

In light of recent developments such as the COP21 climate agreement, UN adoption of the Sustainable Development Goals for 2030, and the Habitat III Conference, there is increasing recognition of the role of human settlements as key components of both global challenges and also global solutions. Urban sustainability or Sustainable Community Development (SCD) is a holistic approach that integrates social, environmental, and economic considerations into the processes and actions undertaken by communities on their path toward sustainability. It entails progress in all forms of community capital: natural, physical, economic, human, social, and cultural [9]. For this paper we use the terms SCD and urban sustainability interchangeably.

We present an overview of the theories that have influenced urban sustainability theory and practice over time (Sections 2 and 3), and suggest a convergence of urban sustainability agendas with strong potential to contribute to healthy and sustainable communities (Section 4).

2. Historical and Conceptual Overview

The term "sustainable development" (SD) has been criticised as ambiguous and open to contradictory interpretations [10]; in the literature, it is more often referred to as the process, the effort, and activities leading to the end goal of sustainability [11]. "Development" should not be confused with "growth"; while quantitative increases (e.g., in income, population, production, and size) are aptly described as "growth", qualitative changes (e.g., in health, knowledge, quality of life, walkability, and efficient resource use) are more accurately described as "development" [9]. Moreover, sustainable development should not be conceived of as a trade-off between the environment and the economy, since protecting ecosystems and developing sustainably need not mean job loss or economic downturn. It is about a new way of thinking about economic development over the long term: it is about "doing development differently" [9].

In a study of several definitions of sustainability, Berke and Conroy [12] identified four common characteristics: (1) "balance" in integrating environmental, economic, and social aspects; (2) the potential of a system to regenerate (recreate and strengthen itself); (3) the recognition that local systems are part of a global system; and (4) the dynamic and ever-evolving nature of SD. They went on to describe SD as "a dynamic process in which communities anticipate and accommodate the needs of current and future generations in ways that reproduce and balance local social, economic, and ecological systems, and link local actions to global concerns" [12].

In this section we follow the progression from the "big picture" of global sustainability and the UN Sustainable Development Goals to local sustainability and Goal 11 on inclusive, safe, resilient, and sustainable cities. We highlight the importance of local communities in dealing with global sustainability issues and trace the underpinnings of sustainable development theory and practice, as these form the conceptual background of sustainable community development.

2.1. Global Developments

The principal global sustainability challenges in the 21st century, i.e., ecological integrity, social equity and cohesion, and economic prosperity, need to be addressed in an integrated way [9,13]. At the time of the UN Conference on Environment and Development (Rio Earth Summit, 1992), we were witnessing the dawn of more mainstream public awareness about environmental issues, also evident in the adoption of the Agenda 21, a sustainable development action plan for the 21st century [9]. Then, the ingredients for change included awareness and some level of political engagement and environmental initiatives, but not the technical capacity, social understanding, and political will for meaningful, structural change [14]. By the time of the World Summit on Sustainable Development in 2002, there was an increasing sense of crisis, as knowledge about the state of environmental systems showed a continued negative trend and need for urgent action [14].

In April 1987, the United Nations World Commission on Environment and Development, chaired by Gro Harlem Brundtland of Norway, released its much-heralded report, "Our Common Future" [9]. The Brundtland Commission Report showed that the poorest fifth of the world's population had less than two percent of the world's economic product while the richest fifth had 75 percent; and that the 26 percent of the world's population living in developed countries consumed between 80 and 86 percent of non-renewable resources and 34 percent to 53 percent of food products [15]. The report emphasised the principle and imperative of sustainable development, which it defined as "meeting the needs of the present without compromising the ability of future generations to meet their own needs" [16].

The Millennium Development Goals (MDGs), unanimously adopted in September 2000 by the United Nations Member States marked a new era for sustainability at the global level [17]. The MDGs were composed of eight goals, 21 targets, and 60 indicators, and encouraged action by a broad range of stakeholders in developed and developing countries, so as to address the multi-dimensional issue of extreme poverty by 2015. Several of the goals have been achieved, with notable decreases in poverty, mortality, and disease rates in the developing world; however, the MDGs have been criticised as vague and potentially leading to further inequality in an urban context [18,19].

By 2012, when the Rio+20 Earth Summit took place, we find ourselves facing an implementation issue, as communities develop sustainability plans without being able to mobilize citizens and apply a holistic approach to their actions [20]. At that Summit, the post-2015 UN Development Agenda was initiated and, in September 2015, 193 countries adopted the Sustainable Development Goals (SDGs) [21]: 17 goals and 169 concrete targets and indicators aiming to tackle poverty, climate change, and inequality in both developed and developing nations [17]. This agenda is grounded in a holistic view of sustainability and on the significance of the environmental dimension of sustainable development for all SDGs. The acknowledgement of the need for integrated action is also evident in the recent UNFCCC COP21 Paris Agreement to keep the global average temperature "well below 2 °C above pre-industrial levels and to pursue efforts to limit the temperature increase to 1.5 °C above pre-industrial levels" [22].

2.2. The Role of Human Settlements

The increasing recognition of the role of human settlements as key components of both global challenges and global solutions follows naturally the exponential growth of urban population: from 30% of the global population in 1950 to 54% in 2014, and expected to reach 66% in 2050 [23], which would correspond to three times the total global population in 1900. The world's urban areas, occupying 3%–4% of the world's land surface, use 80% of its resources, and discharge most of the planet's solid, liquid, and gaseous waste [24]. At the same time they become increasing vulnerable to climate change risks and, subsequently, face serious health challenges which are in turn linked to extended healthcare, infrastructure, and other costs burdening the economy and the environment [25].

However, communities today "constitute the arena where action is concretized; [...] they are transformative; they [...] are hubs of peer-to-peer learning and knowledge sharing" [26,27]. As early as the Rio Earth Summit in 1992, ICLEI—Local Governments for Sustainability (ICLEI) catalysed the adoption of Local Agenda 21, an initiative promoting a larger role for local authorities in sustainability planning [28]. Twenty years later, the Rio+20 conference encouraged sustainability assessment at the local community level [9]. The current global discussion on local SD solutions, as well as the recent adoption of UN Sustainable Development Goal 11 for "inclusive, safe, resilient, and sustainable" human settlements, again demonstrate the significance of urban sustainability [29]. Local governments are the laboratories for successful, monitorable, and transferable sustainability policies and practices, and quite possibly our best chance to deal with the environmental impact of human activity [17,30].

As governments were beginning to perceive the magnitude and ramifications of rapid urbanisation, the first UN Conference on Human Settlements (Habitat I), was convened in 1976 in Vancouver, Canada [28]. With Habitat III taking place 40 years later in October 2016 in Ecuador, the emphasis is on sustainable urban and territorial development which requires "(1) integrated policy formulation and implementation; (2) transformative renewal strategies; (3) environment planning and management; (4) planning compact and connected cities and regions; and (5) inclusive and participatory planning" [31].

One of the paradoxes related to urban sustainability is directly linked to the plethora of definitions for sustainable development and the various notions attached to it by researchers and practitioners. We want to highlight though that, despite the lack of definitional consensus, SCD, like SD, has three core elements on which researchers and practitioners generally agree: the environment (carrying capacity of the biosphere and resource management), the society (addressing equity, inclusion, cohesion, and poverty), and the economy (qualitative and quantitative economic performance) [9].

2.3. Theories and Factors Influencing Sustainable Community Development over Time

2.3.1. Ecological Modernisation

A key concept that has formed the basis of various environmental or development strategies as well as urban sustainability initiatives over the past two decades is ecological modernisation, which was coined in the 1980s as a response to the environmental degradation apparently due to the relentless pursuit of economic growth [28]. Through improvements in technology and design, energy and resource efficiency, and innovations in production, ecological modernisation primarily seeks to achieve congruence between the economic and the ecological dimensions of sustainability [28].

The ecological modernisation proponents believe that innovation and technology can provide sound solutions to environmental problems created by human activity and at the same time contribute to further growth by turning to a "cleaner" economy that internalizes the environmental risks [32]. This theory, reconciling resource efficiency and business growth, has also been called "a profitable sustainability" [33] and inspired some Northern European countries to develop environmental policies for emissions abatement and eco-efficient production processes in the 1990s [28].

The main debate on ecological modernisation relates to its scope, which is restricted to ecological and economic concerns, thus not incorporating important issues such as social equality, population trends, and inter- and intra-generational equity [28]. Especially in its early steps, ecological modernisation theory was primarily connected to mainstream theories promoting economic growth, such as capitalism and industrialism, and therefore subscribed to weak sustainability principles (see discussion below) [34].

There is also a tendency evident in ecological modernisation to rely on technological advance as the "magic formula" to cure or reverse environmental problems [35]. The persistence of efficiency solutions and technological innovations demonstrates the lack of an integrative approach to current global and local issues that require deeper social change [28,36].

2.3.2. Weak vs. Strong Sustainability

In economics, sustainability is defined in terms of economic growth through the neoclassical production function, a widely used way to calculate economic growth: $Q = Q(K, L)$, where Q is the quantity of economic output, K is capital (composed of human/manufactured capital or K_h and natural capital or K_n), and L is labour. For neoclassical economists, production inputs (K and L) are substitutable. This however is not always the case: a sawmill (manufactured capital) and a forest (natural capital) are not necessarily substitutable, and some natural capital degradation or extinction is unquestionably irreversible [37].

Weak sustainability advocates assume that natural resources are super-abundant or that the elasticity of substitution between K_n and K_h is larger than 1 or that technological progress can increase the productivity of K_n at a faster pace than that of its depletion. They believe in perfect substitution between manufactured and natural capital of equal value, while the total capital stock remains constant [38,39]. Proponents of "weak sustainability" promote an anthropocentric worldview, that humans should dominate over nature and that economic growth (or human welfare) can continue indefinitely [34].

Moving gradually to stronger sustainability has been a subject in SD discussions for the past few decades, as ecological economists such as Herman Daly have argued that natural resources are not substitutable inputs since they are not infinite [6]. *Strong sustainability* holds that the various production inputs should exist independently [40,41] and that in some cases environmental damage and resource depletion cannot be reversed [34]. For strong sustainability advocates, the existing stock of natural capital must be maintained (or even enhanced for the sake of future generations), because the functions it performs cannot be duplicated by manufactured capital. Therefore, ecological sustainability is a prerequisite to economic development (this viewpoint prefers the term "development" over the term "growth", as "development" additionally incorporates social equity and qualitative improvement) [42].

A middle perspective considers only "critical natural capital" (i.e., ecosystem services providing life-support functions) as non-substitutable [43]; it may thus be possible to substitute between forms of Kn that are not "critical" (e.g., raw materials, waste assimilation, and amenities) or when there is a significant benefit from resource depletion or a large cost for conservation [37]. This however assumes complete information about all natural capital and its depletion impact, which is not the case.

Questions that constitute arenas for debate and research in this area relate to how each type of capital can be accurately measured (particularly how to assign monetary values to ecosystem services), whether GDP is a good measure of progress toward sustainability, what measures and indicators can effectively account for resource degradation, social equity, and non-market services, etc. Summing up, strong sustainability seems to be heading in the right direction for SCD: preserving adequate amounts of all natural assets (not constant, because population and other factors change as well) while avoiding terminal damage to critical natural assets, and consciously seeking to address key social issues [9].

2.3.3. Social Economy, Community Economic Development, Green Economy, and Self-Reliance

The social economy discourse emerged as a community response to negative impacts of social and economic restructuring, for instance through free trade agreements and privatisation [44]. Although a number of definitions exist resulting in significant debates, SE generally refers to activities by democratically controlled organisations and associations that integrate a social and economic mission, exist between the private and public sectors, and/or use the market to pursue explicit social objectives [44,45].

The social economy field has evolved rapidly, from simple forms of economic activity reflecting social or cultural values to social and green enterprise ventures. It is estimated that the social economy employs at least 2 million people in Canada and 11 million in the European Union [45]. Some SE initiatives have been criticised for operating inside the capitalist system and therefore by this system's rules instead of trying to change them [14].

Community Economic Development (CED), often considered as a predecessor of the social economy, refers to bottom-up initiatives and participatory processes in which economic activities that meet social needs and environmental well-being are developed [44,45]. Social economy and CED are not completely synonymous; CED is locally focused and emphasizes collective bottom-up action, whereas SE is not necessarily geographically focused and builds on both collective action and individual entrepreneurship [45]. Although social economy and CED mostly combine social and economic aspects of sustainability, they can considerably contribute to local sustainability when converged with SCD, which integrates the environmental dimension along with the other two [44].

Two more concepts are worth briefly mentioning here, as they relate to the social economy and CED discussion: green economy and self-reliance or eco-localism. The Rio+20 process popularised the "green economy", which brings environmental considerations into the social economy and uses the latter to advance equity concerns within sustainability. Related to the debate on weak and strong sustainability, this approach moves along a spectrum between initiatives that are criticised for not addressing societal transformation and those that prioritize equity and social needs over profit maximisation. According to Connelly et al. [14], "a critical point of differentiation is whether social economy/enterprise activities are able to generate their own capital, rather than relying on an ongoing subsidy from the derivatives of the mainstream economy and the politics of redistribution".

Eco-localism integrates social, economic, and environmental sustainability, by focusing on the creation of self-reliant economies at the local level [46]. Through self-reliance initiatives, diversification of local economies is encouraged so that communities meet their needs, foster equity and inclusion, manage energy and waste more efficiently, and become more aware of the environmental and social impacts of economic activities [9]. This approach recognizes that there may be limits to the natural and human capital within and around a given local community, and that the road to self-reliance requires collective agreement, capacity building, and decision-making based on the integrated concept of sustainable community development [46].

2.3.4. Resource Efficiency, Circular Economy, and Urban Metabolism

A further shift in sustainability thinking occurred with key research papers such as that by von Weizsäcker et al. [46], which states that an 80% increase in resource productivity could be achieved through the use of efficient design, technology, and management. Concepts like eco-efficiency, circular economy, and turning waste into resources have resulted in "green" economic and business strategies, called "resource efficient"; businesses have started to adopt such concepts and to use efficient design, technology, and management [47].

Meanwhile, the concepts of urban metabolism and circular economy build upon the perception of a city as an ecosystem in which energy and material are the inputs and wastes are the outputs [48]. Urban metabolism based on a circular economy has been propagated mostly by McKinsey and Company [49] and the World Future Council [24,50]. Studies using urban metabolism principles and metrics have shown the ever-increasing urban demand for natural resources [51] and this finding has formed the rationale for various sustainability and resource efficiency initiatives worldwide [52]. Overall, the above demonstrate an advancement in the environmental-economic dimension of sustainability, by moving from the effort to reduce the global impact of human activity on the environment to the potential of resource efficiency and regeneration, and self-reliance [53].

2.3.5. The "Social" and "Just" Aspects of Sustainability

Despite the existence of various definitions and interpretations of SD and SCD, in most cases the triple bottom line is prominent. From municipal sustainability plans to corporate sustainability reporting, they usually review the environmental, economic, and social dimensions of an activity or initiative. However, they are rarely reviewed with equal attention; the environmental and economic aspects of sustainability are generally more visible than the social aspect.

Social capital can encompass characteristics such as social responsibility, trust, shared knowledge, and norms (cognitive social capital), as well as networks, structures, and relations within and beyond a community (bonding and bridging social capital) [9,37]. It is potentially a public good, usually under-provided by private agents, and exists only when combined with trust, credibility, and reciprocity. In contrast with natural capital, social capital will not be depleted if it is increasingly being used, but will deplete very quickly if it is not used.

Some researchers consider that sustainability is an advancement of the environmental justice movement which emerged in the 1980s through the convergence of social and environmental activism [54,55]. The concept of environmental justice, which could be loosely defined as the right to clean and safe environment for all (or even the fair distribution of the social, cultural, and health impacts of environmental degradation), is critical for the achievement of SD and SCD goals.

Agyeman, Bullard, & Evans [54] explain that the relationship between environmental degradation and social capital, as described above, has three main characteristics: (1) the two aspects are progressing in parallel, in that—at any jurisdictional or geographical level—"human inequality is bad for environmental quality"; (2) environmental problems are incommensurately afflicting the poorest societal groups; and (3) both aspects need to be treated as parts of the holistic approach which constitutes the basis of sustainable development.

As Agyeman indicates [56], even though environmental sustainability is fundamental, the aspects of social equity and welfare have to be integrated with the environmental and economic aspects. He calls this connection "environmental quality-human equality" for present and future generations. Social sustainability then became stronger as researchers (e.g., [56,57]) and citizen movements demanded the inclusion of social concerns, such as intra-generational equity, into any SD discussion. The social dimension of SD has thus been introduced in the literature through concepts such as "environmental justice" [54], "just sustainability" [56] and "shared ethical framework" [58].

2.3.6. Resilience

Although an old concept for engineering, psychology, and disaster management, resilience with regards to ecological and socio-ecological systems was first introduced by the renowned natural scientist C.S. Holling in 1973. A resilient system is characterised by its dynamic nature, multiple stable states, uncertainty, and persistence to exist—even if altered—in face of gradual or rapid change [9,47]. An inclusive definition for resilience is "the capacity of a system to absorb disturbance and reorganize while undergoing change so as to still retain essentially the same function, structure, identity, and feedbacks" [59].

Both in the literature and in practice, sustainability and resilience seem to overlap in that they share some principles and goals. The theme of resilience in the context of cities has proven to be very popular in urban planning. Although there are a variety of definitions for and understandings of resilience in social sciences [60], Meerow et al. (2016) concluded that *urban* resilience has not been comprehensively defined yet, as such a venture requires that resilience thinking takes into account the complexity and dynamics of urban systems. They go on to define urban resilience as "the ability of an urban system—and all its constituent socio-ecological and socio-technical networks across temporal and spatial scales—to maintain or rapidly return to desired functions in the face of a disturbance, to adapt to change, and to quickly transform systems that limit current or future adaptive capacity" [61].

There is also another aspect of resilience that "concerns the capacity for renewal, re-organisation and development, which has been less in focus but is essential for the sustainability discourse...in a resilient social-ecological system, disturbance has the potential to create opportunity for doing new things, for innovation and for development" [62]. Even though adopting strategies for resilience is only a part of SCD policy-making, a city may be resilient not only with regards to a natural disaster, but also when facing economic or social turbulence. It is in this respect that resilience supports the normative nature of sustainability by recognizing that a sustainable society is one that is actively seeking to become a better society [9].

Resilience in urban planning is a key driving principle behind the "Transition Town initiative" that emerged in 2006 in the United Kingdom, in response to rising concerns about climate change and peak oil [63]. By emphasizing the need for local action, the "Transition Towns" movement encourages communities to take steps to reduce carbon emissions, prepare for an economy post-peak oil, and ultimately transition to more sustainable socio-technical systems [9]. Towns across the United Kingdom, Australia, the United States, and many more countries are using this framework to plan for sustainability; as of December 2015, there were 479 transition initiatives underway [64].

2.3.7. The Ecological Footprint

A great influencer of the sustainability assessment literature is the ecological footprint developed by Wackernagel and Rees, which estimates the land area and related natural capital required by any human activity, i.e., the land occupied by buildings or infrastructure and the land needed to produce food and production inputs and to assimilate pollutants [65]. The ecological footprint can offer a meaningful single measure of all global ecological impacts of human activities, at household, municipal, national or global levels. The degree to which the footprint of human activities exceeds the total productive area is a measure of unsustainability [9].

The ecological footprint tool compares human demand for resources to the renewable resources available for consumption, i.e., to the Earth's biocapacity. It estimates the global hectares (gha) necessary for human demand by adding up all of the area required to provide these renewable resources, the area of built infrastructure, and the area needed to absorb waste [66]. In 2011, the Earth's biocapacity was estimated at approximately 12 billion hectares which, if divided by the total population that year (~7 billion), gives 1.72 gha per capita [67]. Advanced technology has expanded the Earth's biocapacity by approximately 13% in the last 50 years, but during the same time the global population increased by around 130%, thus reducing the available biocapacity and raising the ecological footprint per person [68]. With the global human population projected to reach 9.6 billion by 2050 and almost 11 billion by 2100 [69], the amount of biocapacity available per capita will further decline.

In the 1970s, humanity entered a state known as "ecological overshoot" [67]: our annual demand for ecological resources has ever since been greater than what the planet can regenerate in a given year. When our consumption exceeds the ecosystem limits, we are drawing down our natural capital and entering a state of overshoot; in ecological footprint terms, we are then appropriating carrying capacity from "distant elsewheres" [65]. Earth Overshoot Day, calculated by Global Footprint Network, an international think tank focused on helping the human economy operate within Earth's ecological limits, is determined for a given year according to the number of days of that year that Earth's biocapacity suffices to provide for humanity's Ecological Footprint; the remainder of the year corresponds to the global overshoot [68].

While ecological footprints have commonly been used on a country scale, they can also be calculated and applied on a local scale. Human communities demand a high input of resources: the more populous the city and the richer its inhabitants, the larger its ecological footprint is likely to be. Although some developed world communities may appear to be sustainable, analysis of their ecological footprint shows that they appropriate carrying capacity not only from their own rural and resource regions, but also from "distant elsewheres" [9]. Where there is availability of reliable local data, the ecological footprint of a community is based on the bottom-up "component" method which reflects the consumption patterns of the local population [51]. For instance, the City of Vancouver, Canada, used this method to assess options for achieving their Greenest City 2020 goals; the action plan includes a short-term goal to achieve a 33% reduction in the City's ecological footprint by 2020 and a longer-term goal to achieve a 75% reduction by 2050 [70]. A related analysis of Metro Vancouver calculated its total ecological footprint in 2006 as an area around 36 times larger than the metropolitan region itself, and thus showed how far the City of Vancouver still is from the "one-planet living" principle included in its Greenest City Action Plan [51].

The ecological footprint analysis has been widely accepted for its strong scientific foundations and for being directly relevant to everyday life and consumption patterns; it has also been criticised for conceptual and methodological weaknesses, as well as for policy-related ineffectiveness [66]. In any case, this approach confirms that we need to minimize consumption of essential natural capital [66]. The question is how to achieve this in the face of contemporary challenges while maintaining or improving quality of life.

2.3.8. Incorporating Public Health Concerns

Public health is another field that influences sustainability theory, planning, and implementation, as a sustainable community is also a healthy community, reflecting the health of its citizens. A century ago, municipalities were instrumental in improving public health by preventing the spread of disease, then viewed as the main challenge for local government. However, health is influenced by the physical and social environments in which we live and work as well as by interventions from the healthcare system [9].

Since the mid-1980s, municipal governments in Europe and North America have adopted a broader conception of public health. The World Health Organisation recognizes that a healthy community respects the principles of participation, partnership, empowerment, and equity, and promotes comprehensive strategies for a health-supportive environment, a good quality of life, and sustainable community development [71]. The fundamental conditions and resources (social determinants) for health are peace, adequate shelter, education, food, income, a stable ecosystem, sustainable resources, social justice, and equity. Thus, a healthy community not only provides adequate housing that is affordable, secure, and fosters a sense of pride and place—it goes beyond housing to improve citizen health, in an integrated, sustainability-inspired sense.

3. Urban Sustainability Implementation and Assessment Hurdles

3.1. Urban Sustainability Planning and Implementation Gap

In the past three decades, recognition of global and local problems, increase of available data, expertise, and technology, and acknowledgement of the need to take action have led to the development and adoption of numerous urban sustainability plans around the world [20]. Similarly, an increase in the number of urban sustainability networks, during the same period, denotes the desire of local governments to cooperate, exchange knowledge and best practices, and be part of a global SD movement [72].

By signing the Aalborg Charter at the 1st European Conference of Sustainable Cities and Towns, organised by ICLEI in 1994 in the aftermath of the Rio Earth Summit, hundreds of local governments have committed to adopting and implementing Local Agenda 21 (LA21) in the form of their own sustainability action plans integrating participatory processes. LA21s promote multi-stakeholder engagement, ecosystem protection, sustainable urban planning, an holistic sustainability viewpoint, participatory decision-making, and establishment of a monitoring framework [28,73]. In 2002, ICLEI reported that more than 6400 communities around the world had committed to the Local Agenda 21 process by that time [74]; 10 years later, however, less than half of them had actively moved beyond the planning stage [20].

As ICLEI's researchers observe [20], municipalities around the world do not exclusively use the LA21 framework; their plans may be called "sustainable development plans", "sustainability action plans", "local sustainability strategies", "integrated development programmes", etc. For instance, around 25% of Canadian communities have adopted Sustainable Community Plans (SCPs) which encompass economic, ecological, and social goals [30], although not all have put implementation strategies in place due to several reasons: capacity-expertise deficit, inability to comprehend and work with the interdisciplinary nature of sustainability, funding shortage, lack of political will, external circumstances, etc. [75]. This gap between planning and implementation has not been without consequences; lost opportunities to act on sustainability, lack of credibility, and increased public scepticism [9,30].

3.2. Issues in Assessing Healthy and Sustainable Communities

The assessment of plans for healthy and sustainable communities is considered an effective tool that follows implementation in order to gauge their success and measure performance in ecological, social, and economic terms [9]. Successful monitoring and assessment of healthy and sustainable communities entails tackling issues such as stakeholder engagement, place-specific challenges, and agreeing on shared theoretical grounds and practical vision [9]. Bond, Morrison-Saunders, and Howitt [76] identified the main debates currently influencing sustainability assessment: (1) the variety of definitions and interpretations of SD by stakeholders; (2) the importance of context for policy actors to agree upon the meaning, implementation, and assessment of SCD in their own case; (3) the relevance of timescales on which SCD plans are built and of impacts that go beyond political boundaries; (4) the dilemma between a reductionist (few indicators covering a broad range of topics) or a holistic approach (many indicators for comprehensive understanding); and (5) the prioritisation of processes or outcomes or both.

Developing an SCD assessment framework needs to be led by a set of guiding principles such as these: livelihood sufficiency and opportunity, intragenerational and intergenerational equity, precaution and adaptation, and resource maintenance and efficiency [77]. Certainly there is not one set of indicators that is perfect for every policy or project, especially given the complex nature of systems and sub-systems in a city [78]. However at least some criteria need to be met so that indicators can be an effective decision-making tool: relevant and meaningful, measurable and feasible, sufficient, timely and consistent, scale appropriate, participatory, and systemic and flexible/modifying [76,78–80].

SCD assessment contains various challenges and debates, most of which have been described above. At the same time, urban sustainability frameworks constitute a rapidly growing arena worldwide, as a multitude of agendas emerged in the past two decades: cities that are "sustainable", "green", "liveable", "smart", "resilient", "eco", "low carbon", "ubiquitous", etc. [32]. The genesis and evolution of most of these agendas seems to have been influenced by the major underpinnings of SD/SCD, ecological modernisation, and the emerging concept of regenerative development or regenerative sustainability [32].

A study of the related literature [32] showed that "sustainable city" is the most frequently mentioned and centrally placed agenda, followed by terms such as "smart city", "digital city", "eco city" and "green city". Smart city and digital city reflect a weak sustainability approach, because the use of technology is prominent as the obvious way to increase productivity, well-being and wealth; whereas the green or eco-city have gained momentum partly because of the increased awareness of climate change challenges. Amidst this multitude of agendas, it is clear that "sustainable city" has longer history, stronger policy associations, and definitely broader scope, i.e., the triple bottom line notion of sustainability. Contrary to perceptions that are popular among decision-makers, this study indicates that these urban sustainability terms should not be used interchangeably, because, although intertwined, they are grounded on various—not necessarily compatible—theoretical premises [32].

Additionally, in the recent years, public health professionals and activists have developed and promoted a "healthy cities" agenda aiming to integrate health concerns in community planning and development. The objective is to reach improved health outcomes and reduced health care costs through enhanced urban design [49]. Health concerns have also been occasionally incorporated into other urban agendas such as eco-cities, low carbon cities, and resilient cities, for obvious reasons: efforts to reverse environmental degradation, maintain ecological integrity, or sustain a status quo in face of climate or other challenges impact human health directly or indirectly [9,32].

The Leverhulme International Research Network *"Tomorrow's City Today: An International Comparison of Eco-City Frameworks"* looked closely at the various existing frameworks developed to assess urban sustainability. In the Network's final report, 43 internationally visible and replicable frameworks are identified and studied; most frameworks (34) have been launched since 2008 and that, contrary to what would be expected, only eight of them have been designed and/or promoted by governmental organisations [81]. The analysis suggests that the vast majority of SCD assessment frameworks fall under one of three broad categories in terms of purpose and usability in decision-making: (1) performance assessment; (2) certification, accreditation or endorsement; and (3) acting as a "planning toolkit" [81].

Joss et al. [81] observe that the 43 frameworks studied by the Leverhulme Network range from focused and minimal to broad and comprehensive sets of indicators (reductionism versus holism) and this often relates to the wide variations noticed in defining and interpreting urban sustainability. The question of process versus outcomes is also tackled in this report, but in conjunction with another dilemma, that of standardisation versus contextualisation. Standardizing sustainability assessment offers advantages such as common language, however urban sustainability is context-specific by nature; keeping this last point in mind may be the key to developing comprehensive frameworks that honour decision-making and participatory process while achieving set sustainability goals. At the intersection of standardisation and contextualisation, it may be helpful to consider indicator frameworks as "boundary objects", i.e., tools that can help operationalize SD and SCD across different policy boundaries [82].

The contextual character of SCD is linked to other issues discussed in the sustainability assessment literature today: (1) the difficulty in deciding the scope of a framework due to questions of spatial and jurisdictional boundaries; (2) the complexity in developing or using replicable and comparable frameworks [81]; and (3) the concerns related to accessible, timely, and reliable data. Standardised, out-of-the-box frameworks are usually excessively data-driven and therefore not always scalable and relevant to particular places, since factors related to social values and visions, community development, and culture may disconnect data from reality [83].

The main finding to emerge from the current research on SCD performance assessment is that the field is not yet fully developed. While there are many frameworks in existence, their development appears to be taking place in a haphazard, siloed manner. Most of these frameworks—and the decision-making processes that result from them—fail to acknowledge the importance of several aspects of sustainability: the systemic nature of cities [33], the strong need for integration of human and environmental health interests [84], the "globalizing world" in which resources are produced and consumed in different regions [85], the need for emphasis on social inclusion, equity, constructive societal mobilisation, and security [48]. These concerns are now manifested in the Sustainable Development Goals as well as the demand for strong sustainability approaches and a common language between sustainability researchers and practitioners and among policy-makers themselves [86]. It is evident, then, that sustainability frameworks need to be enhanced and possibly aggregated [81,87] so as to promote healthy community capital management and regeneration.

3.3. The Community Capital Framework

The Community Capital framework [9] and the tools that have been developed to operationalize it constitute an inspiration for our research in exploring the advancement of SCD planning and assessment. We use the term "Community Capital" (Figure 1) to include natural, physical, economic, human, social, and cultural forms of capital.

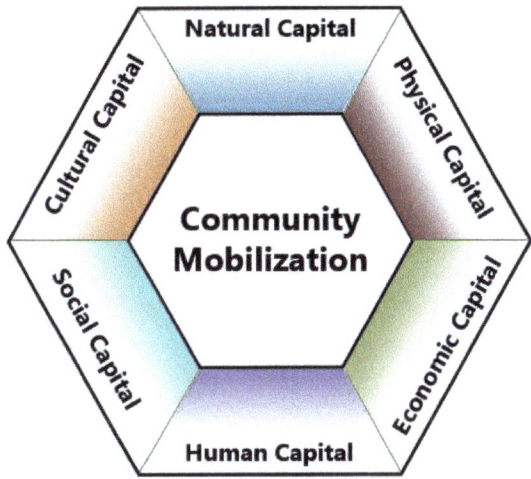

Figure 1. *Community Capital: A Framework for Sustainable Community Development.* Sustainable development requires mobilizing citizens and their governments to strengthen all forms of community capital. Community mobilisation is necessary to coordinate, balance and catalyze community capital. Source: [9].

(1) *Natural Capital:* Minimizing the consumption of essential natural capital means living within ecological limits, conserving and enhancing natural resources, using resources sustainably (soil, air, water, energy, and so on), using cleaner production methods, and minimizing waste (solid, liquid, air pollution, and so on).

(2) *Physical Capital:* Improving physical capital includes focusing on community assets such as public facilities (e.g., hospitals and schools), water and sanitation provision, efficient transport, safe and high-quality housing, adequate infrastructure, and telecommunications.

(3) *Economic Capital*: Strengthening economic capital means focusing on maximizing the use of existing resources (using waste as a resource, for example), circulating dollars within a community, making things locally to replace imports, creating a new product, trading fairly with others, and developing community financial institutions.

(4) *Human Capital*: Increasing human capital requires a focus on areas such as health, education, nutrition, literacy, and family and community cohesion, as well as on increased training and improved workplace dynamics to generate more productive and innovative workers; basic determinants of health such as peace and safety, food, shelter, education, income, and employment are necessary prerequisites.

(5) *Social Capital*: Multiplying social capital requires attention to effective and representative local governance, strong organisations, capacity-building, participatory planning, and access to information as well as collaboration and partnerships.

(6) *Cultural Capital*: Enhancing cultural capital implies attention to traditions and values, heritage and place, the arts, diversity, and social history [9].

The Community Capital Tool (CCT) is an SCD assessment tool built upon the Community Capital framework, and is the product of collaboration between the Centre for Sustainable Community Development at Simon Fraser University in Canada, with Telos, Brabant Center for Sustainable Development, Tilburg University, Netherlands. The six capital accounts of the CCT are broken down into a set of smaller stocks and requirements used to measure capital capacity and sustainability progress. The stocks are subsystems that influence the state and development of each capital account and can be considered as assets. These stocks are, for the most part, universal and were chosen based on their ability to accurately and efficiently represent the health of the capital they represent. Within each stock is a set of requirements that are chosen by the community to more closely represent the local needs and priorities of the community or of the specific initiative being measured. Lastly, each requirement is measured by one or more indicators. Indicators are specific, measurable entities (such as GHG emissions, unemployment rates, etc.) that "indicate" the status of each requirement. They are selected based on the ease (and cost) of their data collection, their correlation to the requirement being measured, and the reliability and integrity of their data sources. The CCT then rolls up the final results into a graphical reporting package that reports on the health of each capital account and each of their constituent stocks. Community leaders, planners, and citizens can use this information to compare the current sustainability status of their community with past results, and with other, comparable communities. The CCT was designed based on strong sustainability principles. It focuses on the issues specific to each individual community, but does so in a way that recognizes each community's regional and global impact on the environment and on society at large. The CCT is also designed to incorporate the democratic input of citizens in terms of values and priorities, and provides planners and decision-makers with a tool that helps them ensure that these values and priorities are reflected in their policy decisions [9].

Of course, the Community Capital Framework and Tool is only one of many frameworks and tools that have been developed to help plan for and assess sustainability; some present conceptual similarities [81] but most come from a variety of theoretical backgrounds [88], while almost all face practical challenges and limitations, as discussed in the previous section. Examples of other significant sustainability assessment frameworks include STAR Community Index, BREEAM Communities, One Planet Communities, the Foundation for Sustainable Area Development method, the Canadian Index of Wellbeing, and Vancouver Foundation Vital Signs.

4. Converging Urban Agendas for Healthy and Sustainable Communities

4.1. Introduction

As human settlements continue to grow and extract resources, they impose a "disproportionate" impact on the biosphere while suffering from economic and social issues within their boundaries [48]. We suggest that another transition, from a negative individualistic logic (reducing impact) to a positive systemic one (regeneration of resources) is imperative; a shift during which community, people, and environment not only coexist but are involved in a co-evolutionary process [89]. As explained above, the triple bottom line perception of sustainability has evolved over the last decades, resulting in a number of agendas which have not always involved a balanced approach between environmental, economic, and social concerns [32,53].

As SCD researchers and practitioners become more aware of planetary ecological constraints combined with urban population and economic growth, they increasingly recognise the significance of urban assets. Traditional economic growth, based on weak sustainability principles, urges cities to maintain or increase their economic output by improving technology, accumulating capital, and enhancing labour productivity. However, urban space that is planned using strong sustainability principles can lead to increases in human, resource, and process productivity, improved urban assets performance, ecological function regeneration and efficient use of resources [49,90].

Urban areas may not be indefinitely sustainable if they continue to be extractive and not productive—it is the potential of advancing SCD through this concept of productivity that our current research explores. With this paper, we seek to advance the big picture—not necessarily by advocating for a new paradigm but by pointing toward a new direction that has the potential to offer a shared understanding. We introduce here our research on productive sustainability, an enhanced SD planning and assessment framework based on strong sustainability principles, aiming to operationalize SD that can successfully address issues of ecological integrity, social equity and cohesion, and economic prosperity.

4.2. Urban Productivity and Regenerative Sustainability

Neo-classical economics defines productivity as a function of labour and capital inputs. Theory has evolved to concepts such as Total Factor Productivity (TFP), which includes more types of input because a "significant" percentage of output could not be attributed to the neoclassical labour and capital inputs [35]. Around the 1980s and early 1990s, the TFP theory included the input of natural resources, policies, knowledge sharing, collaboration, and expertise, while in the 1990s it came to serve as the basis of local and regional economic development strategies, along with other concepts such as ecological modernisation, circular economy, cluster development, and innovation strategy [49]. These concepts and strategies resulted in the emergence of a wide range of urban development agendas as described above; agendas promoted by various actors and networks, oftentimes with the ambition to address social, environmental, and economic issues simultaneously, albeit usually without much success.

Drawing from these agendas, the limited regenerative or productive sustainability literature, and the realities of the 21st century, we argue that a productive city would seek to regenerate its resources, by being net-positive, i.e., producing more capital than it consumes [33,50,91]. What would a regenerative or productive city entail? Reduced ecological footprint, efficient renewable energy systems, regenerating soils with organic matter, replenishing plant nutrients, regenerating forests, restoring watersheds [24], regenerative water supplies, renewed human connection with nature, expanded green economy, increased livability, innovation, social inclusion, and participatory decision-making [86].

Productivity is multi-dimensional, in the same way as sustainability [92]; full productivity potential can only be achieved through a holistic approach, which integrates economic, social, and environmental factors and their myriad interconnections [93]. Enhancing productivity therefore entails investment and improvements at least in the following capitals: social (connectedness, tolerance, inclusion), human (knowledge, skills, health), physical (infrastructure, technology), and economic (financial and business resource allocation) [9,49].

The interdisciplinary nature of the productivity concept has the potential to offer the common language and the long-term and comparative perspective needed for SCD planning and assessment [86]. The increase of productivity at the local level requires the collaboration among all interested actors and can offer opportunities that have not been explored yet, for economic activities and new markets, employment and social inclusion, as well as preservation of the natural environment [52].

Productivity is a notion that resonates with people simply because it is relevant to everyday life; therefore it has potential for greater uptake than concepts such as sustainability that seem more abstract (particularly while researchers and practitioners still seek consensus on their definitions) [94]. Additionally, economic productivity is a quite developed concept in terms of theory and practice and it can be combined with functional definitions of social and environmental productivity in order to advance our understanding and implementation of sustainability.

The concept of productivity may also be seen as related to the perception of sustainability as a process; as Neuman and Churchill [95] explain, sustainability should be studied as applying in complex open systems and in life-cycle processes, since this is the way to go beyond "sustaining" the resources and reach "rates of production and regeneration that equal or exceed rates of consumption and by-product absorption". This perspective incorporates a dynamic approach to production and consumption which is present in the—new and modest—literature on urban productivity or regenerative sustainability [48,91,96], as well as applying the laws of thermodynamics to urban systems which may have unclear boundaries. So, "what kind of city would we have if its assets, systems, and places were simultaneously competitive, livable, just, healthy, sustainable, smart, resilient, regenerative, safe, creative, and happy? In short..." a productive city [49].

Examples of small-scale productive or regenerative community initiatives can be found within municipalities such as Adelaide, Australia (efficient use of local resources, dynamic public consultations, major organic waste composting schemes, and impressive renewable energy development), and Copenhagen, Denmark (energy efficiency initiatives, public transit and cycling uptake, extensive information campaigns and debates, and exemplary waste management) [24]. Regenerative practices also exist around the world in the realm of sectoral policies such as energy (e.g., Beddington Zero Energy Development (BedZed) in the United Kingdom,

Masdar in Abu Dhabi, Portland's Eco-District initiative, the Arbed scheme in Wales, United Kingdom, or districts in Frieburg and Hamburg, Germany), and agriculture (e.g., urban farming programmes in Havana, Cuba, community gardens in New York City and elsewhere, or energy efficient and hydroponic use of farmland in Shanghai and Beijing, China) [9,24,97].

4.3. Healthy and Productive Communities

We need to move beyond initiatives that focus on only one or two dimensions of SD and work toward communities that explicitly integrate ecological, economic, and social sustainability principles and practices. We showed above that health is directly related to the holistic notion of sustainability—but how is health related to productivity?

Improving productivity in the workplace is not a new concept, but in the 20th century it was almost exclusively associated with economic growth, i.e., the increase of economic output and profit for a given organisation or economy [98]. This led industrialised countries, such as the United States, to "overwork" their labour force at the expense of their well-being, as manifested in recreational time, health, and activities strengthening social interactions [99].

Observing weak sustainability principles, technological innovation would replace human labour and enhance productivity, however history has showed that this has not been the case in some developed countries, where longer hours of work were required for growth despite post-World War II technological advances [100]. Seen, however, through a strong sustainability lens, the increase of labour productivity, which is often demanded today due to the pressure to lower labour cost, does not need to involve longer work hours or further technological innovation to replace human labour. More hours of work are not necessarily followed by proportional increases in productivity or prosperity as expressed by income [101].

In the modern economy, productivity should increase output through enhanced labour force [98] and healthier work and life conditions, while reducing the use of natural resources [102]. Improving work and life productivity that encompasses the principles of social equity and social inclusion has the potential to contribute to reversing the decline of social capital and contribute to healthier communities [37,99]. Investment in labour productivity, by creating opportunities for education, training, and employment for marginalised or less-favoured people, has beneficial effects on a community's health and mobilisation of social capital [37]. Investment in place-based productivity (in the workplace, in the community, at home, etc.) is associated with improved physical and mental health, higher performance, more robust personal relationships, continuous learning, and adaptation and sense of belonging [49,103].

5. Conclusions and Further Research

We have shown above that the concept of sustainability has evolved from an effort to reduce the impact of human activity on the environment [37] to the potential of regeneration [36] and self-reliance [104], as viewed from a strong sustainability perspective [5,14]. Human settlements today generally extract resources at a rate faster than the biosphere can replenish; if this model continues, the natural ecosystem is at risk of collapse [85]. Since cities continue to grow while both reducing the biosphere's carrying capacity and suffering from economic and social issues, a shift in the sustainability paradigm is required. While a sustainable (net-zero) city focuses on limiting its ecological footprint and applying social considerations in the economy, a productive (net-positive) city would regenerate its resources by producing more than it consumes and by replenishing its capital from within.

The interdisciplinary nature of productivity has the potential to offer common language, shared understanding, and long-term perspective for SCD planning, implementation, and assessment. Current theoretical approaches and practical applications of environmental or economic productivity are not necessarily intertwined at the local level; in particular, most do not yet seem to adequately encompass social productivity. Local productivity requires multi-stakeholder collaboration and inclusion of social considerations, and thus can offer opportunities that have not before been fully explored.

Our current research involves the development of an analytical conceptual framework, drawing from a detailed literature review on urban productivity and regenerative sustainability. The focus then will center on testing the concepts and measures of economic, ecological, and social productivity in the urban context, through the application of the urban productivity framework on case studies in Canada. During this research we will utilize "Pando | Sustainable Communities", www.pando.sc, a web-based, multilingual, and fully-featured collaboration platform designed as a place for sustainability researchers and practitioners globally to meet, share ideas and work towards common SD and SCD goals [72]. Through the Pando network we will both disseminate our work and invite colleagues around the world to pilot our framework with communities in their own countries. By testing the urban productivity framework in as many communities as possible, we aim to improve its relevance, usability, and potential to provide much-needed integrated local solutions to global challenges. This research will aid in demonstrating whether a focus on converging these urban agendas, through a focus on community capital productivity and regeneration, may be the key to advancing healthy and sustainable communities.

Acknowledgments: We appreciate Jeb Brugmann and the members of the Urban Productivity Collaborative (via Pando) for inspiring and encouraging our interest in urban productivity and regenerative sustainability.

Author Contributions: The authors contributed equally to this work. Both authors read and approved the final manuscript.

Conflicts of Interest: The authors declare no conflict of interest.

References and Notes

1. Hodson, Mike, and Simon Marvin. "Urbanism in the anthropocene: Ecological urbanism or premium ecological enclaves?" *City* 14 (2010): 298–313.
2. Steffen, Will, Åsa Persson, Lisa Deutsch, Jan Zalasiewicz, Mark Williams, Katherine Richardson, Carole Crumley, Paul Crutzen, Carl Folke, Line Gordon, and et al. "The anthropocene: From global change to planetary stewardship." *Ambio* 40 (2011): 739–61.
3. Meadows, Donella H., Dennis L. Meadows, Jorgen Randers, and William W. Behrens. *The Limits to Growth*. Washington: Club of Rome, 1972.
4. Meadows, Donella H., Dennis L. Meadows, and Jørgen Randers. *Beyond the Limits: Global Collapse or a Sustainable Future*. London: Earthscan Publications Ltd., 1992.
5. Hamstead, Meredith P., and Michael S. Quinn. "Sustainable Community Development and Ecological Economics: Theoretical Convergence and Practical Implications." *Local Environment: The International Journal of Justice and Sustainability* 10 (2005): 141–58.
6. Daly, Herman E. "Economics in a Full World." *Scientific American* 293 (2005): 100–7.
7. Steffen, Will, Katherine Richardson, Johan Rockström, Sarah E. Cornell, Ingo Fetzer, Elena M. Bennett, Reinette Biggs, Stephen R. Carpenter, Wim de Vries, Cynthia A. de Wit, and et al. "Planetary boundaries: Guiding human development on a changing planet." *Science* 347 (2015): 1259855.
8. Rockström, Johan. "A safe operating space for humanity." *Nature* 461 (2009): 472–75.
9. Roseland, Mark. *Toward Sustainable Communities: Solutions for Citizens and Their Governments*, 4th ed. Gabriola Island: New Society Publishers, 2012.
10. United Nations Department of Economic and Social Affairs. *Sustainable Development Scenarios for Rio+20. A Component of the Sustainable Development in the 21st Century (SD21) Project*. New York: United Nations Department of Economic and Social Affairs, 2013.
11. Sartori, Simone, Fernanda Latrônico, and Lucila Campos. "Sustainability and Sustainable Development: A Taxonomy in the Field of Literature." *Ambiente & Sociedade* 17 (2014): 1–20.
12. Berke, Philip R., and Maria Manta Conroy. "Are We Planning for Sustainable Development?" *Journal of the American Planning Association* 66 (2000): 21–33.
13. International Council for Science (ICSU), and International Social Science Council (ISSC). *Review of Targets for the Sustainable Development Goals: The Science Perspective*. Paris: ICSU, 2015.
14. Connelly, Sean, Sean Markey, and Mark Roseland. "We Know Enough: Achieving Action Through the Convergence of Sustainable Community Development and the Social Economy." In *The Economy of Green Cities*. Dordrecht: Springer, 2013, pp. 191–203.

15. World Commission on Environment and Development. *Report of the World Commission on Environment and Development: Our Common Future (The Brundtland Report)*. New York: WCED, 1987.
16. United Nations. "Report of the World Commission on Environment and Development—Our Common Future. Annex to Document A/42/427." 1987. Available online: http://www.un-documents.net/wced-ocf.htm (accessed on 2 October 2015).
17. Woolbridge, Michael. *From MDGs to SDGs: What Are the Sustainable Development Goals?* Bonn: ICLEI—Local Governments for Sustainability, 2015.
18. Harcourt, Wendy. "The Millennium Development Goals: A missed opportunity?" *Development* 48 (2005): 1–4.
19. Meth, Paula. "Millennium development goals and urban informal settlements: Unintended consequences." *International Development Planning Review* 35 (2013): v–xiii.
20. Rok, Ania, and Stefan Kuhn. *Local Sustainability 2012: Taking Stock and Moving Forward—ICLEI Global Review*. Bonn: ICLEI, 2012.
21. United Nations. *Resolution 70/1. Transforming our World: The 2030 Agenda for Sustainable Development*. New York: United Nations, 2015.
22. United Nations. *Adoption of the Paris Agreement (FCCC/CP/2015/L.9/Rev.1)*. Paris: United Nations, 2015.
23. United Nations Department of Economic and Social Affairs. *World Urbanization Prospects: The 2014 Revision, Highlights (ST/ESA/SER.A/352)*. New York: UNDESA, 2014.
24. Girardet, Herbert. "Creating Regenerative Cities." Available online: http://www.sustainable-performance.org/wp-content/uploads/2013/10/Regenerative-Cities.pdf (accessed on 12 September 2015).
25. Harlan, Sharon L., and Darren M. Ruddell. "Climate change and health in cities: Impacts of heat and air pollution and potential co-benefits from mitigation and adaptation." *Current Opinion in Environmental Sustainability* 3 (2011): 126–34.
26. United Nations. *The Future We Want (Resolution Adopted by the General Assembly on 27 July 2012) (A/RES/66/288)*. New York: United Nations, 2012.
27. UNDESA. *World Economic and Social Survey 2013*. New York: UNDESA, 2013.
28. Bayulken, Bogachan, and Donald Huisingh. "A literature review of historical trends and emerging theoretical approaches for developing sustainable cities (part 1)." *Journal of Cleaner Production* 109 (2015): 11–24.
29. Kanie, Norichika, Naoya Abe, Masahiko Iguchi, Jue Yang, Ngeta Kabiri, Yuto Kitamura, Shunsuke Mangagi, Ikuho Miyazawa, Simon Olsen, Tomohiro Tasaki, and et al. "Integration and Diffusion in Sustainable Development Goals: Learning from the Past, Looking into the Future." *Sustainability* 6 (2014): 1761–75.
30. Cairns, Stephanie, Amelia Clarke, Ying Zhou, and Vincent Thivierge. *Sustainability Alignment Manual (SAM)*. Ottawa and Waterloo: Sustainable Prosperity and University of Waterloo, 2015.
31. UN HABITAT. *International Guidelines on Urban and Territorial Planning: Towards a Compendium of Inspiring Practices*. Nairobi: UN HABITAT, 2015.

32. De Jong, Martin, Simon Joss, Daan Schraven, Changjie Zhan, and Margot Weijnen. "Sustainable-smart- resilient-low carbon-eco-knowledge cities; making sense of a multitude of concepts promoting sustainable urbanization." *Journal of Cleaner Production* 109 (2015): 25–38.
33. Du Plessis, Chrisna. "Towards a regenerative paradigm for the built environment." *Building Research & Information* 40 (2012): 7–22.
34. Williams, Colin C., and Andrew C. Millington. "The Diverse and Contested Meanings of Sustainable Development." *The Geographical Journal* 170 (2004): 99–104.
35. Burkett, Paul. "Total Factor Productivity: An Ecological-Economic Critique." *Organization & Environment* 19 (2006): 171–90.
36. Reed, Bill. "Shifting from 'sustainability' to regeneration." *Building Research & Information* 35 (2007): 674–80.
37. Roseland, Mark. "Sustainable community development: Integrating environmental, economic, and social objectives." *Progress in Planning* 54 (2000): 73–132.
38. Solow, Robert M. "An almost practical step toward sustainability." *Resources Policy* 19 (1993): 162–72.
39. Ayres, Robert U. "On the practical limits to substitution." *Ecological Economics* 61 (2007): 115–28.
40. Ayres, Robert U. "Eco-thermodynamics: Economics and the second law." *Ecological Economics* 26 (1998): 189–209.
41. Ayres, Robert U. "Sustainability economics: Where do we stand?" *Ecological Economics* 67 (2008): 281–310.
42. Bartelmus, Peter. "The future we want: Green growth or sustainable development?" *Environmental Development* 7 (2013): 165–70.
43. Neumayer, Eric. "Human Development and Sustainability." *Journal of Human Development and Capabilities* 13 (2012): 1–19.
44. Gismondi, Mike, Sean Connelly, Mary Beckie, and Mark Roseland. *Scaling Up*. Athabasca: Athabasca University Press, 2016.
45. Hernandez, Gretchen. "From Spaces of Marginalization to Places of Participation—Indigenous Articulations of the Social Economy in the Bolivian Highlands." Ph.D. Thesis, Simon Fraser University, Burnaby, BC, Canada, 14 May 2015.
46. Von Weizsäcker, Ernst, Karlson Hargroves, Michael Smith, Cheryl Desha, and Peter Stasinopoulos. "Chapter 1—A Framework for Factor Five—The Natural Edge Project." In *Factor 5: Transforming the Global Economy through 80% Increase in Resource Productivity—A Report to the Club of Rome*. London: Earthscan Publications Ltd., 2009.
47. Hodson, Mike, and Simon Marvin, eds. *After Sustainable Cities?* Abingdon, Oxon and New York: Routledge, 2014.
48. Newman, Peter, and Isabella Jennings. *Cities as Sustainable Ecosystems: Principles and Practices*. Washington: Island Press, 2008.
49. Brugmann, Jeb. "The Urban Productivity Imperative." In *The Productive City: Growth in a No-Growth World (Pre-Publication Draft)*. Toronto: The Next Practice Ltd., 2015.

50. Girardet, Herbert. "Sustainability is Unhelpful: We Need to Think about Regeneration." *Guardian*, 10 June 2013. Available online: http://www.theguardian.com/sustainable-business/blog/sustainability-unhelpful-think-regeneration (accessed on 3 November 2015).
51. Moore, Jennie, Meidad Kissinger, and William E. Rees. "An urban metabolism and ecological footprint assessment of Metro Vancouver." *Journal of Environmental Management* 124 (2013): 51–61.
52. OECD. *OECD Green Growth Studies: Material Resources, Productivity and the Environment*. Paris: OECD, 2015.
53. Brugmann, Jeb, and Eugene Mohareb. "The Productive City: Defining the practices of urban ecological development." Paper presented at the 8th World Congress of ICLEI—Local Governments for Sustainability, Belo Horizonte, Brazil, 14–17 June 2012.
54. Agyeman, Julian, Robert D. Bullard, and Bob Evans. "Exploring the Nexus: Bringing Together Sustainability, Environmental Justice and Equity." *Space and Polity* 6 (2002): 77–90.
55. Salcido, Rachael E. "Reviving the Environmental Justice Agenda." *Chicago-Kent Law Review* 91 (2016): 115–37.
56. Agyeman, Julian. "Toward a 'just' sustainability?" *Continuum: Journal of Media & Cultural Studies* 22 (2008): 751–56.
57. Agyeman, Julian. *Introducing Just Sustainabilities: Policy, Planning, and Practice*. London and New York: Zed Books, 2013.
58. The Earth Charter Initiative. *The Earth Charter*. Ciudad Colón: The Earth Charter Initiative, 2010.
59. Walker, Brian, Crawford S. Holling, Stephen R. Carpenter, and Ann Kinzig. "Resilience, Adaptability and Transformability in Social-Ecological Systems." *Ecology and Society* 9 (2004): 5.
60. Olsson, Lennart, Anne Jerneck, Henrik Thoren, Johannes Persson, and David O'Byrne. "Why resilience is unappealing to social science: Theoretical and empirical investigations of the scientific use of resilience." *Science Advances* 1 (2015): e1400217-1-11.
61. Meerow, Sara, Joshua P. Newell, and Melissa Stults. "Defining urban resilience: A review." *Landscape and Urban Planning* 147 (2016): 38–49.
62. Folke, Carl. "Resilience: The emergence of a perspective for social-ecological systems analyses." *Global Environmental Change* 16 (2006): 253–67.
63. Baker, Susan, and Abid Mehmood. "Social innovation and the governance of sustainable places." *Local Environment: The International Journal of Justice and Sustainability* 20 (2013): 321–34.
64. Transition Network. Available online: https://www.transitionnetwork.org/ (accessed on 3 November 2015).
65. Wackernagel, Mathis, and William E. Rees. *Our Ecological Footprint*. Gabriola Island: New Society Publishers, 1996.

66. Rees, William E. "Ecological footprints and biocapacity: Essential elements in sustainability assessment (Ch 9)." In *Renewables-Based Technology: Sustainability Assessment*. Edited by Jo Dewulf and Herman Van Langenhove. Chichester: John Wiley and Sons, 2006.
67. McLellan, Richard, Leena Iyengar, Barney Jeffries, and Natasja Oerlemans. *WWF Living Planet Report 2014: Summary*. Gland: World Wide Fund, 2014.
68. Ecological Footprint Network. Available online: http://www.footprintnetwork.org/en/index.php/GFN/ (accessed on 3 November 2015).
69. UNDESA. *World Population Prospects: The 2015 Revision, Key Findings*. New York: UNDESA, 2015.
70. City of Vancouver. "Greenest City 2020 Action Plan." 2012. Available online: http://vancouver.ca/files/cov/Greenest-city-action-plan.pdf (accessed on 3 November 2015).
71. World Health Organization. "WHO Healthy Settings Programme." Available online: http://www.who.int/healthy_settings/en/ (accessed on 3 November 2015).
72. Roseland, Mark, and Freya Kristensen. "Mobilising collaboration with Pando|Sustainable Communities." *Local Environment: The International Journal of Justice and Sustainability* 19 (2014): 469–78.
73. Clarke, Amelia. "Key structural features for collaborative strategy implementation: A study of sustainable development/local agenda 21 collaborations." *Management & Avenir* 50 (2011): 153–71.
74. ICLEI—Local Governments for Sustainability. "Second Local Agenda 21 Survey, Background paper No. 15." 2002. Available online: https://divinefreedomradio.files.wordpress.com/2013/10/sustainabledevelopment2nd-prepsession.pdf (accessed on 3 November 2015).
75. Clarke, Amelia. *Passing Go: Moving Beyond the Plan*. Ottawa: FCM, 2012.
76. Bond, Alan James, Angus Morrison-Saunders, and Richard Howitt. *Sustainability Assessment. Pluralism, Practice and Progress*. Abingdon, Oxon and New York: Routledge, 2013.
77. Gibson, Bob, Selma Hassan, James Tansey, and Graham Whitelaw. *Sustainability Assessment: Criteria and Processes*. Abingdon, Oxon and New York: Routledge, 2005.
78. Meadows, Donella H. *Indicators and Information Systems for Sustainable Development*. Hartland: The Sustainability Institute, 1998.
79. UN SDSN. "Indicators and a Monitoring Framework for Sustainable Development Goals—Launching a Data Revolution for the SDGs." 2015. Available online: http://unsdsn.org/resources/publications/indicators/ (accessed on 12 September 2015).
80. Henderson, Nancy. "Measuring Up." *The Social Planning and Research Council of BC News*. 2006. Available online: http://www.sparc.bc.ca/resources-and-publications/doc/242-article-measuring-up-sparc-bc-news-nancy-henderson-v23-no1-winter-2006.pdf (accessed on 15 November 2015).
81. Joss, Simon, Robert Cowley, Martin de Jong, Bernhard Müller, Boom Soon Park, W. Rees, Mark Roseland, and Yvonne Rydin. *Tomorrow's City Today: Prospects for Standardising Sustainable Urban Development*. London: University of Westminster, 2015.

82. Holden, Meg. "Sustainability indicator systems within urban governance: Usability analysis of sustainability indicator systems as boundary objects." *Ecological Indicators* 32 (2013): 89–96.
83. Kitchin, Rob. "Making sense of smart cities: Addressing present shortcomings." *Cambridge Journal of Regions, Economy and Society* 8 (2015): 131–36.
84. Secretariat of the Convention on Biological Diversity. *Cities and Biodiversity Outlook: A Global Assessment of the Links between Urbanization, Biodiversity, and Ecosystem Services*. Montreal: Secretariat of the Convention on Biological Diversity, 2012.
85. Kissinger, Mark, and William E. Rees. "Assessing Sustainability in a Globalizing World." *Journal of Industrial Ecology* 13 (2009): 357–60.
86. Roseland, Mark. "Growth, Prosperity and Jobs for all, Within Planetary Boundaries (Final Issues Paper)." 2014. Available online: http://communitascoalition.org/pdf/Final_Urban_Prosperity_Roseland.pdf (accessed on 20 January 2014).
87. Joss, Simon, and Daniel Tomozeiu. *"Eco-City" Frameworks—A Global Overview (Survey Conducted as Part of The Leverhulme International Network "Tomorrow's City Today)*. London: University of Westminster, 2013.
88. Tanguay, Georges A., Juste Rajaonson, Jean-François Lefebvre, and Paul Lanoie. "Measuring the sustainability of cities: An analysis of the use of local indicators." *Ecological Indicators* 10 (2010): 407–18.
89. Neuman, Michael. "The Compact City Fallacy." *Journal of Planning Education and Research* 25 (2005): 11–26.
90. Girardet, Herbert. *Creating Regenerative Cities*. Abingdon, Oxon and New York: Routledge, 2015.
91. Robinson, John, and Raymond J. Cole. "Theoretical underpinnings of regenerative sustainability." *Building Research & Information* 43 (2015): 133–43.
92. World Confederation of Productivity Science. Available online: http://www.wcps.info/ (accessed on 10 November 2015).
93. Burgess, Thomas F., and John Heap. "Creating a sustainable national index for social, environmental and economic productivity." *International Journal of Productivity and Performance Management* 61 (2012): 334–58.
94. Berke, Philip R. "Does Sustainable Development Offer a New Direction for Planning? Challenges for the Twenty-First Century." *Journal of Planning Literature* 17 (2002): 21–36.
95. Neuman, Michael, and Stuart W. Churchill. "A general process model of sustainability." *Industrial & Engineering Chemistry Research* 50 (2011): 8901–4.
96. UBC. "UBC Centre for Interactive Research on Sustainability—Regenerative Neighbourhoods Program." Available online: http://cirs.ubc.ca/research/research-portfolio/regenerative-neighbourhoods (accessed on 29 August 2015).
97. Hunt, Miriam, and Carla De Laurentis. "Sustainable regeneration: A guiding vision towards low-carbon transition?" *Local Environment: The International Journal of Justice and Sustainability* 20 (2015): 1081–102.
98. Jackson, Tim, and Peter Victor. "Productivity and work in the 'green economy'." *Environmental Innovation and Societal Transitions* 1 (2011): 101–8.

99. Putnam, Robert D. "Bowling Alone: America's Declining Social Capital." *Journal of Democracy* 6 (1995): 65–78.
100. Schor, Juliet B., and Dennis Chamot. "Workers of the world. Unwind." *Technology Review* 94 (1991): 24.
101. Knight, Kyle W., Eugene A. Rosa, and Juliet B. Schor. "Could working less reduce pressures on the environment? A cross-national panel analysis of OECD countries, 1970–2007." *Global Environmental Change* 23 (2013): 691–700.
102. Davies, John. "The Ecological Footprint, Sustainability and Productivity." *Management Services* 52 (2008): 35–40.
103. Jackson, Tim. *Prosperity without Growth?—The Transition to a Sustainable Economy*. London: Sustainable Development Commission, 2009.
104. Curtis, Fred. "Eco-localism and sustainability." *Ecological Economics* 46 (2003): 83–102.

A Case Study in Organizing for Livable and Sustainable Communities

Jerry Marx and Alison Rataj

Abstract: Citizens in the U.S. are making organized efforts to demand a new approach to planning urban communities, one that results in more sustainable and livable communities. The profession of social work in the U.S. once had a primary role in organizing urban residents to advocate for healthier environments in their neighborhoods. Yet, recent research documents the diminishing emphasis on community organization as an intervention method in social work. This paper offers a descriptive case study of a successful community organizing effort to promote a more livable city in Portland, Maine (USA). Data was collected by the authors using in-depth personal interviews; archival records (census data, architect models); documents (e-mails, newspaper clippings) as well as direct observation of the impacted community and development site. Implications for social work practitioners and educators involved in community organization promoting healthy communities are presented.

Reprinted from *Soc. Sci.* Cite as: Marx, J.; Rataj, A. A Case Study in Organizing for Livable and Sustainable Communities. *Soc. Sci.* **2016**, *5*, 1.

---

1. Introduction

Community organization as an intervention method in the profession of social work has a long history. Beginning in the late 1800s, social workers, nurses, and others, established nonprofit organizations called "settlement houses" in poor, inner-city neighborhoods to improve the living conditions of recent immigrants. As such, they served as vehicles for documenting the needs of community residents, organizing community services, and advocating for a healthier neighborhood environment. "Residence, research, and reform" summed up the strategy of settlement leaders, who lived in the neighborhood settlements along with recent immigrants, documented health risks, and then lobbied city government and corporations for change [1]. Public meetings, lectures, group discussion, neighborhood surveys, and direct observation were the primary communication and data collection methods employed by settlement leaders and residents. Social work pioneers, such as Jane Addams, were leaders in the settlement house movement, thereby establishing community organization as a fundamental intervention method in social work.

Recent research, however, documents the diminishing emphasis on community organization in professional social work [2,3]. There are several factors that contribute to this trend, including the lack of community organization skills among social work educators and diminishing community organization content in the social work curriculum [4]. Social work has survived as a profession in part because of its broad applicability in an ever-changing world. If community organization is to survive as a social work intervention method, then a broader, more contemporary conceptualization of community organization is needed—one that utilizes the latest technologies to address current public concerns about livable communities.

Research in this area, particularly on the use of digital technologies in community organization as well as other types of civic and political participation, is just emerging and has shown mixed results [5–9]. With the premise that "communities" should be broadly defined as groups of people who form a distinct social unit based on location, interests, or identification, this paper offers a descriptive case study of a successful community organizing effort to promote a more livable city in Portland, Maine (USA). In so doing, the case illustrates new motivations, tactics, and technologies for community organization in social work. Data was collected by the authors using in-depth personal interviews; archival records (census data, architect models); documents (e-mails, newspaper clippings) as well as direct observation of the impacted community and development site [10].

2. The Case of Portland, Maine

Portland is located on the southeastern seaboard of Cumberland County in the state of Maine—about an hour drive north of Boston, MA. Once known for its manufacturing, shipping and industrial production, Portland now specializes in tourism, education and health services [11]. If its suburbs are excluded, this small city is home to 66,214 people, yet has 16 distinct neighborhoods [12]. Portland has seen a surge of urban development to accommodate an anticipated population growth as the Boston metropolitan region spreads northward up the coastline. Given it location, Portland ranked as the nation's 43rd largest hotel market, and attracted 8.1 million visitors in 2012, with tourists spending an estimated $4.1 billion in one year [13].

However, there is another side of Portland. According to 2012 census data in Portland, 19.4% of individuals are below the federal poverty level. Finding apartments to rent in Portland has become a challenge for low and moderate income residents as well as individuals looking to relocate to the city. Vacancy rates dropped from 7.5% to approximately 2% over the last five years. The average monthly rent for a two-bedroom apartment has risen from $850 in 2010 to over $1050 [14]. Even though Portland boasts 17,000 rental units, more than half (58%) of Portland residents are renters, meaning that these properties are insufficient to meet a growing demand for rental units. What is more, with 1502 houses or condos per square mile, there is not much more room to develop in the city. To partially address this need, the City of Portland made plans to add 190 market-rate units to be built by a Miami-based developer in the city's Bayside neighborhood. The city and the developer argued that this project is crucial to the city's future [15,16]. One group of concerned neighborhood activists disagreed.

3. A Victim of Urban Renewal

The neighborhood of Bayside is situated midway on a city peninsular that runs from Portland's scenic eastern neighborhood of Munjoy Hill to its fashionable "West End" neighborhood. The decline of the Bayside neighborhood began in the 1970s, when the city tore down buildings in the neighborhood to make way for the Franklin Arterial. While making it easier for suburban commuters, this highway effectively dissected the Bayside neighborhood into two parts, isolating one part of the community from the other by creating a barrier to walkability. Since then, the city has been attempting to redevelop the neighborhood but has consistently denied proposals. In 2000, the city planning department issued the "Bayside Vision", which called for more housing and larger, taller buildings in the area, including the former scrapyard in the center of the neighborhood. The plan also recognized a related need for a city-funded parking garage. In July 2011, the city agreed to sell 3.25 acres in Bayside to an out-of-state developer, Federated Companies, for $2.3 million, with an agreement that any development would include a parking garage paid for in part with $9 million in federal money passed through the city. In the fall of 2012, Federated unveiled their $105 million dollar plan, subsequently referred to as the "Midtown Project" [17].

4. New Urban Planning Theory

From January 2013 until April 2013, the city held workshops on the proposed Midtown development, where "Keep Portland Livable", a group of community residents, business owners, and activists, vehemently opposed it. Based on the latest thinking in urban planning theory, the group maintained that this development would not promote a livable community. Contemporary urban planning theory has its origins in the activism and writing of Jane Jacobs, who argued that "urban renewal" was destroying the livability of urban neighborhoods. Based on her observations in Boston's North End neighborhood, New York City's Greenwich Village, and elsewhere, Jacobs argued that healthy urban communities with vitality contained densely populated neighborhoods involving short city blocks; mixed land uses (residential, business, *etc.*), moderately high buildings of 4–5 stories, wide sidewalks catering to pedestrians, and centrally-located parks [18]. The city of Portland has become highly attractive because it meets these characteristics. Jacobs was scoffed at by city officials and urban planners in her time, but many eventually agreed with her critique. Consequently, her theory and vision have remained highly influential in urban planning, inspiring the "New Urbanism" movement in the housing development industry [19–22].

In contrast, the Midtown development, argued neighborhood activists, was repeating the urban renewal mistakes of the past. The project would be out of scale with the building heights of the neighborhood, and with its proposed parking garages, overly auto-centric, paving the way for more cars to enter the city at the expense of residents and pedestrians. Consequently, Keep Portland Livable clashed with the city council, which held the belief that a new large-scale housing development would cure the housing crisis. Further, the state laws of Maine do not allow city taxes, so the city of Portland is heavily dependent on property taxes. One way to raise funds, therefore, is to push out nonprofits, and bring in big developments. This combined with the project's now archaic use of urban design would lead to negative consequences for the city of Portland, argued Keep Portland Livable. More precisely, opponents warned that the developer's proposal featured high rise towers that would destroy site lines, cast significant shadows, and generate dangerous wind tunnels. In addition, the project lacked sufficient open space and sidewalks [22].

With respect to building height, according to city building code regulations in Bayside, buildings are not to exceed the zone's current 125-foot height limit; the new development's height, however, would need to be 165 feet. Consequently, in April of 2013, the Portland City Council voted to grant a building height exemption for the massive project. Prior to the meeting, Keep Portland Livable published an advertisement in the city's major newspaper, the Portland Press Herald, alerting the public to the mammoth size of the proposed project and to the fact that the City Council would be voting to grant a height exemption. At the City Council Meeting on 22 April 2013, after having spent thousands of dollars to run the awareness ad, only a handful of people showed up to support Keep Portland Livable. Consequently, the Portland City Council approved the zoning height amendment [23].

After the zoning decision, Keep Portland Livable realized that the city wanted this project to move forward, regardless of existing city regulations. These community activists knew they would need sophisticated support to effectively oppose the development. Consequently, in April 2013, Keep Portland Livable retained a land-use attorney who attended all of the future city planning board workshops related to the Midtown project. Then, in August 2013, the group hired a communications consultant to aid in public relations, media campaigns and awareness strategies.

With the support of their communications consultant, in September of 2013, Keep Portland Livable hired a polling firm, Public Policy Polling, to conduct a 500-person phone poll of Portland residents regarding the Midtown project. Results showed that after completing the questionnaire, 30% of respondents were in favor of the development, 54% were opposed, and 16% were unsure. Given this documentation of public opposition, the group's lead organizers decided to increase their advocacy efforts [22].

In October of 2013, Keep Portland Livable publicly launched its website, Facebook page, LinkedIn and Twitter accounts. The group's leaders used technology as a strategy to help build stronger public opposition to the Bayside project. In addition, the organizers reached out to friends and affiliates to pitch in and show up at meetings. They developed list of names of Bayside residents and potential donors, then e-mailed letters to these people about the Bayside project. As a result, Keep Portland Livable began to see a steady increase in supporters.

The group also mounted a media campaign in which it sent out press releases to TV stations, public radio and newspapers. Furthermore, the leaders of Keep Portland Livable scheduled informal house parties where they presented a PowerPoint slideshow about the problems surrounding the Midtown Project. Since all neighborhoods in Portland have a neighborhood organization, they were able to meet with community residents from all parts of the city in hopes of mounting a rally of support [24].

The first planning board public hearing was scheduled for December 2013. Keep Portland Livable began to ready their constituents by sending out flyers and talking points. Additionally, up to this point, the developer had gotten away without showing any images of what the towers would look like. To address this, Keep Portland Livable hired an architect to make digital renderings, using Google Earth, of what these towers would actually look like in Portland. The group then had these images printed and put on large easels right as people walked into the planning board meeting. Their strategy worked. At the first planning board public hearing, the council chambers were packed with a big turnout of Midtown opponents.

The second planning board public hearing was scheduled for January 2014. In a classic trick, the developer packed the council chambers early in the day with construction workers from around the region. Nonetheless, there was still a strong turnout from the opponents of the Bayside Project, who were educated and prepared with more talking points. However, the opposition was not enough and the planning board approved the Bayside project [23].

On 12 February 2014, Keep Portland Livable announced its legal appeal to the planning board approval of the Midtown Project. Grounds for the appeal centered on the project's failure to comply with the city's comprehensive plan and land use ordinances as well as the lack of planning board authority to approve the more than 20 significant waivers granted from city standards and codes. This opposition and advocacy by Keep Portland Livable effectively slowed the development process to a halt, giving time for other Portland residents and business owners to realize the project's full implications. Fearing rising construction costs, mounting citizen anger, and the ultimate demise of its project, Federated Companies, the Miami development company, in October of 2014, conceded to the community activists' demands and pledged to work with Keep Portland Livable and the city to lower the height and general scale of the project along the lines proposed by Keep Portland Livable. More specifically, the plan was scaled back from its original proposal for two 14-story towers and two parking garages. The revised proposal involved four six-story buildings and just one parking garage [23]. As it turned out, the community organizers and supporters of Keep Portland Livable proved that you can fight city hall.

5. Conclusions

The case of Portland's Bayside neighborhood and Keep Portland Livable provides several important lessons for social worker practitioners and educators involved in community organization, and specifically, the promotion of healthy communities.

5.1. Keep Portland Livable Was a Technological Movement

The group's lead organizers made effective use of new technologies to rapidly mobilize opposition to the Midtown project as originally designed. Given that the group, Keep Portland Livable, did not exist before the Midtown project was announced, organizers were able to quickly educate and mobilize Portland residents by constructing a website (700 signups for updates and action alerts), establishing a Facebook page (525 likes), and a Twitter account (over 100 followers). E-mail and LinkedIn were also used extensively. In a small city, this level of community participation is significant [25].

The effectiveness of using Facebook and other new technologies such as Twitter to organize social action activities has been demonstrated by the Occupy Wall Street movement and public protests against police violence in U.S. minority communities. Given this track record and appeal to young people, such technologies need to be emphasized as part of community intervention methods in social work education and utilized extensively by social workers in community organizing.

5.2. Keep Portland Livable Represented an Online Community

It can be argued that Keep Portland Livable was, to a large extent, a "community" based on location. Yet, although the Bayside neighborhood was the battlefront for community organizers, the community residents that followed and supported this organizing effort actually resided in various neighborhoods of Portland as well as outlying suburbs. They did not represent the traditional case of neighbors living on the same street or block or even same neighborhood. For example, the community organization model often used in traditional social work education is Jane Addams and Hull House, which was an inner-city settlement house strategically located within walking distance of the train station in the midst of a poor immigrant neighborhood in Chicago. As previously described, community organizers resided in the settlement house, which, in turn, was the primary vehicle for communication and organizing. Most community discussion took place at this meeting place in the neighborhood.

In contrast, Keep Portland Livable was not a traditional geographic community of neighbors helping neighbors, but, more accurately, an online community of shared vision and values. Most communication and organizing were done electronically. Many members of Keep Portland Livable had witnessed the mistakes of traditional urban planning, whether in Portland or elsewhere, and therefore, subscribed to the promise and values inherent in contemporary urban planning theory and its vision of healthier cities. What is more, it is argued here that a broader conceptualization of community, one that transcends geographic location, to emphasize shared vision and values involving what characterizes healthy community environments, enhances the opportunity for attracting support (volunteers and donations) from outside the community. In this digital advocacy age, that support can extend worldwide.

5.3. Keep Portland Livable Reflected a Desire for a Greener, Sustainable Community

This shared vision of the community organizers, as stated, was for a more sustainable, livable community. The prevention of global warming and preserving a healthy environment are increasingly primary interests of the general public, and, therefore, represent a core issue for future community organization by social workers and others. In fact, concern for the environment is a tradition in Maine, given its economic dependence on natural resources [26]. Research has shown that the "greenest" communities are densely populated urban areas where dwellings are built vertically, recreation areas are shared by many, and residents use bicycles, public transportation, or their legs for commuting [27]. The Midtown project, particularly as envisioned by community activists in this case, promotes these characteristics.

5.4. Keep Portland Livable Was a Network of Professional Specializations

The core group of community organizers in this case was actually small. Although it began with several people, the driving force behind the organizing effort consisted of just two concerned Portland residents, a local architect and an organizational development consultant. However, Keep Portland Livable was able to raise funds to hire several other specialized professionals as needed. As stated earlier, the group enlisted the services of a land-use attorney to attend city Planning Board meetings. This helped to better inform public opposition to the project, counter the technical expertise of Portland's city government, and provide credibility to the group's effort. In addition, Keep Portland Livable hired a communications consultant and polling consultants to assist with a media campaign, surveys, and other public education strategies. Furthermore, Keep Portland Livable hired an architect to make digital renderings, using Google Earth, of what the proposed Midtown project towers would actually look like in Portland. The group displayed these graphic images on its website and at city planning board meetings. The lesson for future community organization is that neighborhood organizations and activist groups should not rely just on community volunteers in order to prevent or promote community change. The technical expertise of those in power needs to be matched to the fullest extent by community residents and organizers. Sometimes, neighborhood volunteers can supply this expertise, but, at times, professionals need to be enlisted.

This study is limited by its single-case design. The authors encourage further case studies of successful community organizing to promote sustainable, livable communities. Such studies might then be generalized in relation to new urban planning theory. More importantly for social work, this research would also serve to inform macro social work education as well as social workers engaged in community organization.

Acknowledgments: The authors would like to acknowledge the contributions to this paper of community organizers Tim Paradis and Peter Monro.

Author Contributions: Both authors contributed equally to this manuscript.

Conflicts of Interest: The authors declare no conflict of interest.

References

1. Jerry D. Marx. *Social Welfare: The American Partnership*. Boston: Allyn & Bacon, 2004.
2. Robert Fisher, and Danielle Corciullo. "Rebuilding community organizing education in social work." *Journal of Community Practice* 19 (2011): 355–68.
3. Jack Rothman. "Education for Macro Intervention: A Survey of Problems and Prospects." *ACOSA*, 2012. Available online: https://www.acosa.org/joomla/pdf/RothmanReportRevisedJune2013 (accessed on 21 December 2015).
4. Shane R. Brady, and Mary Katherine O'Connor. "Understanding how community organizing leads to social change: The beginning development of formal practice theory." *Journal of Community Practice* 22 (2014): 210–28.
5. Shane R. Brady, Jimmy A. Young, and David A. McLeod. "Utilizing digital advocacy in community organizing: Lessons learned from organizing in virtual spaces to promote worker rights and economic justice." *Journal of Community Practice* 23 (2015): 255–73.
6. Sujin Choi, and Han Woo Park. "An exploratory approach to a Twitter-based community centered on a political goal in South Korea: Who organized it, what they shared, and how they acted." *New Media & Society* 16 (2014): 129–48.
7. Sanne Kruikemeier, Guda van Noort, Rens Vliegenthart, and Claes H. de Vreese. "Unraveling the effects of active and passive forms of political Internet use: Does it affect citizens' political involvement? " *New Media & Society* 16 (2014): 903–20.
8. Daniela V. Dimitrova, Adam Shehata, Jesper Stromback, and Lars W. Nord. "The effects of digital media on political knowledge and participation in election campaigns: Evidence from panel data." *Communication Research* 41 (2014): 95–118.

9. Terri L. Towner. "All political participation is socially networked? New media and the 2012 election." *Social Science Computer Review* 31 (2013): 527–41.
10. Robert K. Yin. *Case Study Research: Design and Methods*, 4th ed. Thousand Oaks: Sage Publications, 2009.
11. Charles S. Colgan. *The Maine Economy: Yesterday, Today and Tomorrow*. Portland: Brookings Institution Metropolitan Policy Program, University of Southern Maine, 2006.
12. U.S. Census Bureau. "State and County Quick Facts: Portland (City) Maine, 2014." Available online: http://quickfacts.census.gov/qfd/states/23/2360545.html (accessed on 6 June 2014).
13. Steve Law. "More Tourists Put Portland at Top of Travel Plans. 2014." Available online: http://portlandtribune. com/pt/9-news/208913-65990-more-tourists-put-portland-at-top-of-travel-plans (accessed on 6 June 2014).
14. Randy Billings, and Staff Writer. "Rental Demand in Portland is through the Roof. 2013." Available online: http://www.pressherald.com/2013/04/28/rental-demand-in-portland-is-through-the-roof_2013-04-29/ (accessed on 11 June 2014).
15. City Data. Portland, Maine. Available online: http://www.city-data.com/city/Portland-Maine.html (accessed on 11 June 2014).
16. Keep Portland Livable. About Us. Available online: http://keepportlandlivable.com/About_us.html (accessed on 6 June 2014).
17. Randy Billings. "Portland Approves $105 Million 'Midtown' Project. 2014." Available online: http://www.pressherald.com/2014/01/14/portland_ approves__105_million__midtown__project_/ (accessed on 6 June 2014).
18. Jane Jacobs. *The Death and Life of Great American Cities*. New York: Random House, 1961.
19. Leigh Gallagher. *The End of the Suburbs: Where the American Dream Is Moving*. New York: The Penguin Group, Inc., 2013.
20. New Urbanism. "Creating Livable Sustainable Communities (2013). 2013." Available online: http://www.newurbanism.org/ (accessed on 6 June 2014).
21. Ruth Fincher. "Urban redevelopment in Boston: Rhetoric and reality." In *Conflict, Politics and the Urban Scene*. Edited by Kevin R. Cox, and Ronald John Johnston. New York: St. Martin's Press, 1982.
22. Peter Monro. "Bayside Vision *vs.* Midtown." *Keep Portland Livable*, 2014.
23. David Carkhuff. "Midtown project in Bayside scaled down, per settlement." *The Portland Sun*, 24 October 2014. Available online: http://www.portlanddailysun.me/index.php/newsx/local-news/ 13150-midtown-project-in-bayside-scaled-down-per-settlement (accessed on 21 December 2015).
24. Keep Portland Livable. "Threats Foreseen to Portland's Ideal Future. 2015." Available online: http://keepportlandlivable.com/threats-foreseen-to-portlands-ideal-future/#more-674 (accessed on 29 August 2015).
25. Tim Paradis, and (Keep Portland Livable, Portland, ME, USA). Personal communication, 30 December 2014.

26. Colin Woodward. *The Lobster Coast: Rebels, Rusticators, and the Struggle for a Forgotten Frontier*. New York: Penguin Group, 2005.
27. David Owen. *Green Metropolis: Why Living Smaller, Living Closer, and Driving Less Are the Keys to Sustainability*. New York: Penguin Books, 2009.

Hybridity: A Theory of Agency in Early Childhood Governance

Rachel Robinson

Abstract: Contemporary social science research concerning governance tends to take an institutional perspective that privileges structural analysis. The resulting body of literature has an emphasis on classification, typologies and regimes. This approach has been criticized on the basis that it neglects the role of agency and context when research concerns complex and heterogeneous community governance cases. An emerging literature on hybridity in social services aims to address the limitations of structural accounts by acknowledging that diverse logics, ideas, and norms influence the way community based social services resist or adapt in turbulent policy environments. This article considers the strengths and limitations of hybridity in development of a research framework incorporating structure, agency and ideas. The relevance of hybridity theory for the Kids in Communities study—an Australian research project investigating neighborhood influences on child development across multiple case study sites—is evaluated.

Reprinted from *Soc. Sci.* Cite as: Robinson, R. Hybridity: A Theory of Agency in Early Childhood Governance. *Soc. Sci.* **2016**, *5*, 9.

---

1. Introduction

The Organization for Economic Cooperation and Development (OECD) recently released its fourth report into quality in early childhood education and care—Starting Strong IV—with the starting line that "Early childhood education and care (ECEC) remains high on the policy agenda in many OECD countries" ([1], p. 13). The interest in early childhood across liberal economies has been prompted by a comprehensive body of research about the impact of early childhood experiences for the life course [2–6]. In Australia, the early childhood sector involves a multitude of complex and often historical governance and service arrangements and is currently the subject of significant policy interest and reform. A key initiative has been delivery of the Australian Early Development Census (AEDC) in 2009, 2012 and 2015. The AEDC is a population measure of early child development, collected on school entry involving a teacher-completed checklist for all children in the first year of school. Results are reported at the neighborhood level across five developmental domains and are intended for use by all levels of government and community to inform policy and practice [1].

Overall, the AEDC data conform with expected patterns between neighborhood demographics and child development outcomes [7]. However, small area data facilitates identification of outlier communities where children are faring better or worse than expected compared with the population socio-demographic profile [8]. The Kids in Communities Study (KICS) aims to investigate these neighborhoods. *Governance* and *services* are two of the five socio-environmental factors (or domains) hypothesized as influencing child development for the purposes of the KICS research [9]. The governance domain considers contextual and local governance factors and the service domain considers quality, access and participation. The KICS research will ultimately be shared amongst communities, local governments and policy makers to inform policy and for use in measuring and improving child development outcomes.

This paper focuses on the intersection of governance and service factors, aiming to draw together data "in order to investigate, or to identify, key factors that seem to have some bearing on an outcome of interest" ([10], p. 70). It is hypothesized that local governance is a factor influencing service quality and access in early childhood education and care (ECEC) and that this, in turn, has a bearing on child outcomes. A multi-case approach has been selected to consider the hypothesis. Cases have been selected on the basis that outliers may provide theoretical insights that are useful for policy in light of the large-N analysis of the population data [11,12].

This paper aims to describe the governance of ECEC services in Australia, specifically in the state of Victoria, and reflect on options for guiding the research approach in case communities. In order to provide insight on the intersection of the governance and service factors, a robust framework for research into community governance is required. The framework needs to accommodate the complexity and heterogeneity of the governance and service factors in the reform environment. The paper aims to consider the strengths and limitations of three waves of governance theory and the relevance of the alternative provided by the emerging hybridity approach when it comes to researching governance of ECEC services in a complex policy environment.

The paper concludes with a suggested framework for research that draws heavily on hybridity as a way of resolving tension between structural and agential accounts where there is dynamic interaction between markets, hierarchies, and networks, and the development of unique third sector arrangements to manage competing logics in social service delivery.

2. Policy Context: Early Childhood Education and Care in Victoria

In Victoria, ECEC is delivered in a range of formats, funded by federal, state and local levels of government and provided by a plurality of organizations involving cooperatives, associations, church groups, local government, private schools, public schools and small owner-operated and large corporate for-profit organizations. The sector is highly heterogeneous, involving a diverse range of service-based, advocacy, professional and member organizations. There are two key funding formats for early years: long day care with a focus on education and care that supports workforce participation; and kindergarten (also known as preschool) with a focus on educative programs in the year before school. The core funding for participation comes from federal and state government and is directed to accredited services through a family entitlement. Where other funding is provided (e.g., for capital works) this is often only available to not for profit cooperatives and associations.

There are over 1200 services in Victoria whose primary mode of service is long day care and a similar number with the primary mode of kindergarten, operators of these services vary in size from providing one service to 173 services [13]. Across Australia, the bulk of ECEC operators (83%) provide only one service [14]. Nearly all ECEC services receive the bulk of their total revenue from governments and this poses interesting questions for complexity and the levels of "public-ness" and "market-ness" across the for-profit and not-for-profit providers in the sector [15].

Kindergartens—particularly those in established urban areas—often have a history dating back many decades, are run by parent committees and benefit from cash or in-kind contributions from local government. Many services were formed in response to perceived welfare needs in the early part of the 20th century or post-war period, and the sector has a strong professional identity. Since the early 2000s, Kindergarten Cluster Management—where Victorian government funding is provided for group employment and management arrangements—is available in recognition of the complexity and resource constraints facing Kindergarten parent committees.

Long day care settings also have a strong tradition of community management, mainly dating from the 1970s when federal funding programs were available to not-for-profit services only. Commercial providers entered the long day care sector in large numbers from 1991 when federal arrangements shifted to demand based funding directed to services through family entitlements. The funding model—which guarantees funding for well over 50% of service costs in advance of providing the service—proved attractive to commercial providers and the number of for-profit providers has grown rapidly since this time [16].

The early 2000s saw a significant expansion of services, dominated by a single corporate provider and this raised concerns about vertical fragmentation, quality, expenditure of public funds and equitable supply emerged [16,17]. These concerns were accompanied by a highly effective narrative about the importance of the early years for brain development and the economic benefit of investing in quality services [2]. In Australia, this was disseminated by influential medical professionals [18] and dovetailed with the government's focus on productivity and female workforce participation. Two key sets of reforms emerged as a result.

The first involved major place-based programs involving cross-sector collaboration and some devolved resource allocation responsibilities. The AEDC was piloted during this time and provided many communities with access to data to engage stakeholders and support decision-making [19]. The second set of reforms addressed fragmentation with legislative changes introducing consistent curriculum, professional, quality and regulatory standards across the range of ECEC settings and jurisdictions in Australia [20,21]. A key development of the reforms was the creation of the statutory Australian Children's Education and Care Authority (ACECQA) governed by a ministerial council appointed board tasked with implementation of the National Quality Framework (NQF). The reforms have created tensions between those that privilege the social justice and child rights perspectives over the economic and productivity perspectives that have been attractive to governments [18,22,23] but are generally agreed to be "bold" and "ambitious" and to raise the bar on access and quality ([24], p. 223).

An outcome of the reforms has been a significant increase in participation and cost and in 2013, the newly appointed Abbott government commissioned a Productivity Commission inquiry into childcare and early learning. The Commission reported in 2015 and the government responded with a "families package". To be implemented from 2017, the package has been criticized for further eroding the idea of ECEC as a community service [25].

Recent reforms in early childhood policy in Australia bring together a range of political, economic and social influences and are the result of a complex interplay of events, relationships, influence and timing [18,26]. From a supra-national perspective, the path to service reform in Australia is unique, the focus has been on quality assurance and there has been a significant investment in measuring child outcomes with the AEDC, but Australia is one of only a handful of OECD nations where there is no statutory entitlement to either a place or free access to early care and education programs before school entry [1].

In communities, ECEC governance has often developed in distinct ways in order to meet specific local needs, and, where they exist, these local models have been both adaptive and resilient in the changing commercial, social and economic environment. The result is a sector that is a mix of interdependent state and non-state arrangements and multi-level governance incorporating membership, advocacy, special interest and professional organizations. Within the sector, there is great diversity, but independent private providers share many qualities with small not-for-profit and community-based providers [16], similarly large not for profit providers and cluster managers may have more in common with corporate providers. All of the organizations have experienced radical change in their operating environments over many years and have adapted in ways that make the traditional classifications of community, market, corporate and hierarchy inadequate. They are influenced by the hierarchical regulatory arrangements, by market arrangements and by their unique history and the communities that use them as well as by each other.

This brief summary of the governance environment for ECEC is intended to provide an introduction to the complexity of community level research given the complex multi-level environment and shifting policy arrangements. The next section considers the relevance of mainstream approaches to governance research in this environment.

3. Governance Research

Governance—a term that has been labeled "promiscuous" and "capacious" [27,28]—is used to describe a shift from centralized to more diffused forms of state power. As well as being loosely defined, a range of terms are related and often used in substitute for one another—for example networks, participation, collaboration, co-production, community decision making. Despite the muddy language, it is generally accepted that key characteristics of governance are "the interdependence of state and non-state actors and institutions in meeting contemporary public policy challenges" ([29], p. 162) and "the exercise of power and the practice of decision making in collective contexts" ([10], p. 68).

Instrumentally, the aim of network governance is to deliver effective decisions and efficient services that reflect the interests of those who participate, but verifying this is challenging with empirical evidence rarely distinguished from "a host of normative assumptions ... embedded in accounts of the benefits of participation" ([30], p. 5).

In response to the complexity of governance research, three "governance schools" have emerged. The first and second of these "waves" focus on institutional–structural analysis regarding the relationship between the policy outcomes and network structures from two contrasting perspectives. The first, which proposed a fundamental shift from government to governance is focused on autonomy in network arrangements independent of markets and hierarchy. The second waves "brings the state back in" and challenges the assumption of a "hollowed out" state with a focus on the changing nature of the "state-society" relationships ([31], pp. 20–22). The third, interpretive perspective, aims to address the limited focus on agency [32].

The Anglo- or first wave governance school assumes a "radical shift from post new public management to network forms of governance" ([33], p. 276) as an alternative to markets and hierarchies. In this approach the focus is on a differentiated polity where the state is hollowed out—replaced by independent, self-organizing networks, with power and influence situated in markets, arm's length agencies and international organizations [34]. The positivist orientation of this school views networks as fixed structures, blurs the distinction between state and society and see actors as rational and motivated by rewards and incentives. The focus of first wave research is on "macro-level questions about the changing role of the state and state-society relations" ([32], p. 196). The network governance approach that accompanies this school assumes "contemporary governance involves negotiations within and between networks, rather than the assertion of authority by government" ([35], p. 35). This shift is contested and "the lack of concern for agency is a well-known criticism of institutionalist approaches" ([33], p. 278) because, as with most institutionalist approaches, it takes a "highly constrained view of agency" based on a "determinist view about the extent to which institutions shape agents" ([36], p. 883).

The second wave of governance theory or the meta-governance school shifts the focus from institutions to structures or from the vertical to the horizontal, this school maintains that while the certainty of traditional hierarchical approaches is lost under governance, the state continues to access policy instruments and wield significant influence to maintain a steering role and dictate "the rules of the game" ([31], pp. 18–19). The focus of research is on concerns of democracy and accountability including the role of interest networks and inclusion and exclusion of actors in networks. In this school, "policy outputs...are the result of actors within structural locations making choices from a range of structurally determined options" ([32], p. 199).

The limitations of the policy network analysis approach that accompanies the second wave concern the lack of "an adequate theory of agency: it is not clear how we explain the role of actors when structures are given such dominance" ([37], p. 762), and "that it does not, and cannot, explain change" [34]. The significance of context may be lost and conclusions drawn without reference to political institutions and norms, for example, "conclusions from research in societies whose governmental norms are consensual is utilized in work on countries with more antagonistic cultures" ([38], p. 605). This approach emphasizes the instrumental contribution of governance, builds patterns and orders that might be difficult to relate to from everyday experience, glosses over the differences between different state structures and struggles to explain change [36].

Emerging from the limitations of the first and second waves, the third wave of governance theory is associated with an "interpretive turn" that is "decentred" and "actor focused" ([34], pp. 1244, 1249). This wave proposes governance can be neither "achieved" nor "mastered" and is not characterized by essential or generalizable properties that transcend the environment in which they arise ([31], pp. 20–22). The third wave of research sees governance as consisting of "contingent practices emerging from different beliefs" ([32], p. 197) and shifts away from the state to focus on individuals, meaning, practices, ideas and games. This approach is associated with constructivist, qualitative and ethnographic approaches to research.

What Are the Problems with These Approaches?

The first and second wave approaches both share a stake in modern empiricism and positivist rational choice approaches, which have led research to "shoehorn" governance cases into categories, potentially confusing ideal types or regimes and the observable characteristics of governance, not to mention as Rhodes does, that these "typologies of networks have become deeply uninteresting" ([34], p. 1249). The critiques of these mainstream approaches tend to concern the inability to explain change; account for the complexity and dynamic permanence of arrangements that don't fit within the hierarchy, network, market triptych; and accommodate questions of agency.

On the other end of the analytical spectrum is the critique that the alternative interpretive approaches rely on agency and discourse at the expense of structure [32,35]. Williams argues that the waves have falsely set structure and agency up as "oppositional" ([39], p. 24) and led to concerns of ontological inconsistencies when it comes to the treatment of social structure, tradition, power and inequality ([32], p. 198). Fawcett and Daujberg ([32], p. 196) suggest the potential for a critical realist approach to address criticisms about the analytical focus on structure.

Hybridity has emerged as an alternative to third wave governance theory. This approach rejects the anti-foundationalist view of the state as hollowed out but incorporates agency and a dynamic relationship between state and society. Associated with this approach is the idea that if "appropriate forms of governance evolve and are performed through the interaction between actors and their context" ([40], p. 125), then there is a need for approaches that: acknowledge the "relational politics of governance" ([41], p. 3); release us from the idea that governance arrangements fit into neat categorizations and universal descriptors [42]; provide a "process-oriented stream of research" ([43], p. 176); accommodate a dynamic and evolving view of the polity; and build on a "convergence between political science and organizational studies" ([34], p. 1258).

4. Conceptualizing Hybridity

In the social sciences, hybrids are arrangements that "mix elements from ... ideal-typical domains" of communities, markets and hierarchies. They are "problematic" arrangements when it comes to research because it is their difference rather than their similarity that brings them together ([44], p. 750).

There are two broad categories of hybrids discussed in the literature, one has emerged as a direct result of the differentiated polity, fragmentation and hollowing out of the state associated with NPM. This includes the privatization of formerly nationalized industries and the creation of quasi-autonomous government organizations [33], operating at arm's length from government, often according to market principles but with regulatory authority or a certain legitimacy regarding (perceived) ties with government. The other is described as a "novel steering mechanism" and involves the "third sector" in a "proliferation of multiple organization networks for delivering public and private goods and services" that challenge the "dichotomy of public/private" ([15], p. 217).

> "Hybrid organizations are multifunctional entities combining different tasks, values and organizational forms. They are composite and compounded arrangements that are combining partly inconsistent considerations producing difficult and unstable trade-offs and lasting tensions". ([45], p. 410)

Analytical approaches to hybrids have tended to view them as fixed structures [15] but more recent literature has shifted from the hybrid hierarchy/market form taken by quasi-government organizations to an interest in the third sector, not for profits and social services. A body of literature has emerged that considers the concept of hybridity to be "under-theorized" and advocates an approach that is more dynamic in acknowledging the plurality of rationalities facing the third sector [42,46]. More recent theory has a focus on social services characterized by interactions between government, business, civil society and not-for-profits. The resulting hybrids have been described as an "inevitable feature of the public sector" and more "chameleons" than "griffins" [44]—that is, their critical characteristic is that they are adaptive to their environment and this leads them to be further described as a "process" and a "kind of coping strategy" [47].

Hybridity in public administration refers to "heterogeneous arrangements, characterized by mixtures of pure and incongruous origins, (ideal) types, 'cultures', 'coordination mechanisms', 'rationalities', or 'action logics'" ([44], p. 750). The key to current thinking is an 'institutional logic perspective', a "meta-theoretical framework for analyzing interrelationships among institutions, individuals and organizations in social systems" ([48], p. 2). It is proposed that this framework has the potential to guide research in multi-level analysis by accommodating the dynamic relationship between individuals, professional groups, organizations and institutions [33,46,49,50].

Friedland and Alford (1991) are credited with initiating the institutional logic approach in response to the perceived limitations of theory regarding the influence of culture and symbols, and contextually parsimonious statements about institutions and institutional behavior. Friedland and Alford describe the "notion of institutional contradiction" as "vital" to meaningful social analysis and argue that institutional logic addresses concerns of theoretical blind spots and "unmapped territory" that appears in pluralist, managerialist and class-theory approaches ([50], p. 241).

Institutional logic nests individuals as agents within systems of organizations and institutions. This perspective—which has traces of Brofenbrenner's [51] ecological systems approach—theoretically constructs the "symbolic world" at the "institutional level" and reconceptualizes institutions as "simultaneously material and ideal, systems of signs and symbols, rational and transrational" ([50], pp. 242–43). Institutional logics—which are named as capitalism, the state, democracy, family, religion and science—are described as "symbolically grounded, organizationally structured, politically defended, technically and materially constrained" as well as being temporally bound ([50], pp. 248–49).

> "Rejecting both individualistic, rational choice theories and macro structural perspectives, they [Friedland and Alford] hypothesized that each of the institutional orders has a central logic that guides its organizing principles and provides social actors with vocabularies of motive and a sense of self". ([49], p. 101)

The institutional logics perspective provides a foundation for three governance configurations: market, hierarchy, and hybrid as an intermediate form [52], although Brandsen, van de Donk and Putters [44] include the informal configuration of family and community in their conceptualization. In theoretical terms, hybrids trade off the price incentives and actor autonomy of market governance for the administrative control and coordination provided by hierarchy and are formal, in contrast to families and communities. Embedded in this understanding is that the hybrid category is capacious, involving a broad spectrum of formal arrangements that are not pure market or pure hierarchy [53].

Agency is fundamental to the hybridity framework because agency is the mechanism for organizational adaptation and resistance, subject to the alternative meanings provided by multiple institutional logics. The implication is that governance is developmental and iterative and comes about as a result of forces exerted by both individuals and institutions. This analytical understanding enables organizations to "conform or deviate from established patterns" and addresses the limitations of governmentality by maintaining that individuals have the agency to "manipulate or reinterpret symbols and practices" ([50], pp. 244, 254) and therefore to internalize and conform to institutional power or to resist change and exert influence.

Hybridity is a useful way to understand social services such as ECEC because "hybridity typically refers to the complex organizational forms that arise as voluntary, charitable, and community organizations confront differentiated task, legitimacy, or resource environments" ([46], p. 433). As discussed above, ECEC services are a diverse and ambiguous mix of state, markets and civil society, this mix of services exerts dynamic influences on each other and distinctions between profit and not for profit providers can become blurred—a quality evident across fields such as health, education and housing [44,54]. Social services embedded in local communities challenge structural analytical approaches because they imply a "world of situated actors whose agency is enabled and constrained by the prevailing institutional logic and who creatively respond by adapting organizational forms to fit the complex environment" ([46], pp. 437, 439).

> "The identification of distinct governance logics is one way of making analytical sense of this diversity whilst recognizing that evolving governance practices may form more context-specific configurations that blend elements of such logics." ([43], p. 177)

How Can Hybridity Tackle Some of the Complexities of Social Services Such as ECEC?

In Australia, ECEC services are subject to distinct governance arrangements, and, despite the current policy interest, there is little social science literature regarding the unique governance environment and mix of provision [55]. The KICS project provides the opportunity to undertake community level research to make sense of local governance and service arrangements and the implications for current and emerging policy priorities. This may include tensions between perceptions of rights, productivity, and quality and child outcomes, particularly in light of contrasting policy approaches in other liberal economies such as New Zealand, Canada and the United Kingdom.

The logics or steering mechanisms of ECEC are described by Brennan *et al.* ([55], p. 378) as:

> "the logic of market provision concerned with profit-seeking through competition; the logic of state provision to meet citizen's social rights operating through formal/public institutions and state bureaucracies; the logic of associations working through formal/private/non-profit bodies whose rules originate in ethical norms and codes; and the logic of informal, private family provision whose rules and practices are embedded in moral/personal obligation and emotional/social relations."

Recent reform in ECEC in Australia also raises the relevance of professional logics [56], particularly their dynamic influence as the sector becomes more highly professionalized as a result of the NQF reforms.

In building a research framework to accommodate change and difference rather than structure and similarity and the relative influence of diverse institutional logics in development of dynamic hybrid forms according to the environment, Denis, Ferlie and Van Gestel [33] offer four "theoretical prisms". These encourage research to "move beyond structural hybridity" and incorporate a dynamic approach that balances micro-, meso- and macro-level approaches and incorporates an integrative multilevel and multi-actor perspective. This approach encourages examination of structures and governance forms and organizational design; institutional dynamics and context; and identities—roles, work practices; and agency and practices.

In addition to these four "theoretical prisms", Skelcher and Smith [46] offer four contextual variables: normative strength; actor identity; value commitment; and environmental turbulence. These variables can help understand unique organizational responses and illuminate trade-offs, adaptations and blockages based on the internal or external environment. The result is that there may be unique expressions of hybridity—"the subjective appreciation of the normative strength of plural institutional logics in a particular context is an important determinant of an organization's response" ([46], p. 445). This understanding leads them to propose five types of organizational hybridity for non-profits—segmented, segregated, assimilated, blended, and blocked [46]. These typologies feel relevant to the mixed arrangements for ECEC and the need for an approach that can support qualitatively diverse governance arrangements across the selected cases for KICS research.

Given that the ECEC sector in Australia is characterized by a range of actors in a dynamic value laden environment which is subject to multiple logics and tensions that may be geographically and temporally specific, these contributions appear more attractive for community case research than the alternative structural approaches. The ethnographic and contextual research methodologies suggested by a hybridity approach are consistent with the selection of geographic cases for the KICS research on the basis of empirical data and acknowledgement that there may be fixed and variable governance factors across the cases.

In order to inform community multi-case research on governance in ECEC services in cases selected on the basis of early child development data, a framework based on the integrative multi-level and multi-actor perspective generated by Denis et al. [33] and incorporating the variables offered by Skelcher and Smith [46] is proposed. This framework is presented in Table 1 with suggested questions and methods.

This table provides a framework for the approach to the research and an overview of possible questions and techniques to interrogate and analyze governance of ECEC services in the KICS case communities where difference and dynamic adaptation is an expected outcome. This framework spans quantitative and qualitative data and accommodates questions of structure and agency as well as conflicting ideas, considerations, demands, structures and cultural elements.

It is anticipated that the framework would provide the basis for questions exploring reforms over the last decade and the complex negotiations that accompany reforms as well as the extent to which macro-narratives are acceptable and can be tailored to the local context. It would be expected that this approach would draw out historical and embedded norms and values, complex sedimentation or layering of structural and cultural features and the extent to which local culture, professional engagement and citizen participation are associated with stable or unstable, coherent or incoherent, shallow or deep hybrids.

Table 1. Theoretical perspectives, questions and methods to interrogate hybridity in kids in communities study (KICS) research.

Theoretical Perspective	Theory (and Level)	What Questions do We Need to Ask to Acquire Relevant Knowledge?	Suggested Methods for KICS Research
Structures or governance forms	Governance theory (Meso)	What are the modes of governance? Who is involved? What is their involvement? What is the mix of governance arrangements? What are the accountability and organisational patterns?	Policy analysis Sector profiles Local profiles Analysis of outcome and quality data
Institutional dynamics	New institutionalism (Macro)	What are the underpinning logics, values and ideology? Do some logics dominate? What are the dynamics of hybridity? Are there ongoing inconsistencies and tensions likely to lead to further change? Is there sedimentation and co-existence of diverse logics? Have archetypes or novel approaches emerged in response to uncertainty or "common enemies"? Are there ongoing cycles of temporary settlement?	Historical analysis Policy analysis Document analysis Elite interviews
Roles and identities	Identity perspective (Micro)	What norms and meaning are assigned to actors in the sector? Are there changing identities? Who is included/excluded? Are there common modes of perception? What are the different identities and narratives? Do professionals engage in active adaptation/resistance? What language and metaphors are used? What stories are told?	Elite interviews Local document analysis Local stakeholder interviews
Agency and practice	Actor network theory (ANT) (Micro)	What are the norms and local stories—who is involved, what do they say, is history important? What is the role of ethical norms and codes? What values, beliefs and meanings are assigned to actors and guide local participation? Are values permanent or shifting, how are values employed in light of "environmental turbulence"? How are contradictions overcome? Are "technologies" employed to hear local voices? Do local networks produce hybrids in action?	Local document analysis Local stakeholder interviews

Adapted from [33,46].

Recently, literature on hybrids has shifted to address the question of how public administrators can "better engage with hybridity as a normal part of everyday practice, rather than to see it as a problem to be overcome" ([53], p. 22). However, this is a complex task, because while the "concept of institutional logics is intuitively attractive, it is arguably difficult to define and ... apply in an analytically useful manner" ([48], p. 1) especially while the concept of "hybridity" within public administration scholarship remains undeveloped [33]. However, while there are some concerns that there is a gap between the theoretical approach and accepted functions of scholarship and policy advice [53], it provides a framework that supports the collection and analysis of nuanced and contextual data and accommodates mixed methods approaches.

> "Hybridity as a transgression of institutional boundaries is thus also intimately connected with hybridity as the construction of a knowledge regime in which every-day, personal and experiential data is valued as much as that collected through quantitative surveys". ([53], p. 19)

The approach to community case research suggested by the "theoretical prisms" and "variables" suggested by Denis, Ferlie and Van Gestel [33] and Skelcher and Smith [46] provides the potential to contribute to knowledge about the interaction of structure and agency in the development of policy, community action and examples of hybridity in practice in the complex and mixed market environment of ECEC governance and services in Australia and contribute to the goals of the KICS project.

5. Conclusions

This article briefly describes the Kids in Communities (KICS) project and the population level data from which case communities have been selected, on the basis that child outcomes deviate from expected patterns. Two of the five socio-environmental factors (or domains) hypothesized as influencing child development for the purposes of the KICS research are described as governance and services.

An outline of the environment in which ECEC governance and service factors interact establishes the complexity and changing shape of the ECEC sector and the historical background and competing logics that have influenced the temporal governance and service arrangements. When considered from a public policy perspective, the sector has followed pathways from benevolent welfare in the first half of the 20th century, centralized planning and funding for not-for-profits in 1970s and 1980s, a shift to demand based funding and market principles in the 1990s, continuing with more hierarchical levers to encourage equitable participation and address issues of fragmentation and accountability in the 21st century. Prospective policy changes and supra-national interest indicate turbulence in this environment is set to continue for some time.

A brief critical review of three waves of governance theory demonstrates that governance scholarship has shifted over time from a focus on structures and the empirical descriptors and typologies of positivist epistemology to decentred accounts with a focus on symbols, values and beliefs. The third wave approach and interpretive methodology provides a useful basis for capturing local knowledge and meaning, but this approach raises methodological concerns for KICS case study analysis. The KICS research aims to examine and identify both common and unique factors that have a bearing on outcomes so they may be shared amongst communities, local governments and policy makers to inform policy and for use in measuring and improving child development outcomes.

The analytical approach provided by hybridity provides a framework that may overcome some of the limitations of structural and interpretive approaches by conceiving the ECEC sector as simultaneously embedded in local individuals, groups, organizations and networks and driven by macro-transformations, economic shifts, and institutional expectations. The framework and questions can accommodate unique and dynamic local governance in the ECEC sector. It enables the co-existence of hierarchical control exerted by the funding and regulatory environment, dynamic interaction between markets, networks and hierarchies and the influence of multiple competing logics that may be expressed in locally unique ways.

On this basis, a hybridity framework has the potential to be valuable for a community study where there is a balance to be struck between micro, meso and macro factors in a constantly shifting service and governance environment. This approach will inform qualitative approaches in the KICS research, and results will be analyzed to consider common factors in case communities and the relevance of the approach for future research, policy and child development outcomes. The KICS project will report on findings in 2016.

Acknowledgments: The author would like to acknowledge the contribution of Doctoral Supervisor Associate Helen Dickinson, School of Government and School of Social and Political Sciences, University of Melbourne and Sharon Goldfeld, Centre for Community Child Health, Royal Children's Hospital, Murdoch Childrens Research Institute and Department of Paediatrics, University of Melbourne. Goldfeld is the Chief Investigator of the Kids in Communities Study.

Conflicts of Interest: The author declares no conflict of interest.

References

1. Organisation for Economic Cooperation and Development (OECD). *Starting Strong IV: Monitoring Quality in Early Chilhood Education and Care*. Paris: OECD, 2015.
2. James J. Heckman, and Dimitriy V. Masterov. "The productivity argument for investing in young children." *Review of Agricultural Economics* 29 (2007): 446–93.
3. Australian Institute of Health and Welfare. *Literature Review of the Impact of Early Childhood Education and Care on Learning and Development: Working Paper*. Canberra: Australian Institute of Health and Welfare, 2015. Available online: http://www.aihw.gov.au/publication-detail/?id=60129552947 (accessed on 4 February 2016).
4. Jack P. Shonkoff, and Deborah A. Phillips. *From Neurons to Neighbourhoods: The Science of Early Childhood Development*. Washington: National Academy Press, 2000.
5. Tim Moore. "Early Childhood and Long Term Development: The Importance of the Early Years (2006)." Available online: https://www.aracy.org.au/publications-resources/command/download_file/ id/97/filename/Early_childhood_and_long_term_development_-_The_importance_of_the_early_years.pdf (accessed on 4 February 2016).

6. Margot Prior, Fiona Stanley, and Sue Richardson. *Children of the Lucky Country? How Australian Society has Turned Its Back on Children and Why Children Matter*. Sydney: Pan Macmillan, 2005.
7. Dan Cloney, Gordon Cleveland, John Hattie, and Collette Tayler. "Variations in the availability and quality of early childhood education and care by socioeconomic status of neighborhoods." Paper presented at International Conference of the Australian Association for Research in Education (AARE) and the New Zealand Association for Research in Education (NZARE), Brisbane, Australia, 30 November–4 December 2015.
8. Robert Tanton, Lain Dare, Ilan Katz, Sally Brinkman, Geoff Woolcock, Billie Giles-Corti, and Sharon Goldfeld. "Identifying off-diagonal communities using the Australian Early Development Census results." *Social Indicators Research*, 2015, in press.
9. Sharon Goldfeld, Geoffrey Woolcock, Ilan Katz, Robert Tanton, Sally Brinkman, Elodie O'Connor, Talya Mathews, and Billie Giles-Corti. "Neighbourhood effects influencing early childhood development: Conceptual model and trial measurement methodologies from the kids in communities study." *Social Indicators Research* 120 (2014): 197–212.
10. Jenny Stewart. "Multiple-case study methods in governance-related research." *Public Management Review* 14 (2012): 67–82.
11. Evan S. Lieberman. "Nested analysis as a mixed-method strategy for comparative research." *American Political Science Review* 99 (2005): 435–52.
12. Bent Flyvbjerg. "Five misunderstandings about case-study research." *Qualitative Inquiry* 12 (2006): 219–45.
13. ACECQA. "National Register." Available online: http://www.acecqa.gov.au/national-registers (accessed on 11 November 2015).
14. ACECQA. "National Quality Framework Snapshot q3 2015." Available online: http://files.acecqa.gov.au/files/Reports/2015/NQF%20Snapshot%20Q3%202015%20FINAL.pdf (accessed on 11 November 2015).
15. Mark A. Emmert, and Michael M. Crow. "Public, private and hybrid organizations: An empirical examination of the role of publicness." *Administration & Society* 20 (1988): 216–44.
16. Deborah Brennan. "The ABC of child care politics." *Australian Journal of Social Issues* 42 (2007): 213–25.
17. Alison Elliott. *Early Childhood Education: Pathways to Quality and Equity for All Children*. Camberwell: Australian Council for Educational Research, 2006.
18. Kathryn Bown. "Insider perspectives on influence and decision making in the Australian political sphere: A case study of national quality policy in ECEC 2006-09." *Australasian Journal of Early Childhood* 39 (2014): 54–63.
19. Centre for Community Child Health. "Australian Early Development Index: Building Better Communities for Children, Evaluation Report." 2007. Available online: http://www.aedc.gov.au/researchers/aedc-research/publications/publication/final-aedi-evaluation-report (accessed on 4 February 2016).

20. Council of Australian Governments. *National Partnership Agreement on Early Childhood Education*. Canberra: COAG, 2008.
21. Council of Australian Governments. *National Partnership Agreement on the National Quality Agenda for Early Childhood Education and Care*. Canberra: COAG, 2009.
22. Deborah Brennan. "Home and away: The policy context in Australia." In *Kids Count: Better Early Childhood Education and Care in Australia*. Edited by Hill Elizabeth, Pocock Barbara and Elliott Alison. Sydney: Unversity of Sydney Press, 2007, pp. 57–74.
23. Eva Cox. "Forget the Productivity Commission. This is What Childcare Should Look Like." *The Guardian Australia Online*, 14 March 2015. Available online: http://www.theguardian.com/commentisfree/2015/mar/14/forget-the-productivity-commission-this-is-what-childcare-should-look-like (accessed on 11 November 2015).
24. Collette Tayler. "Changing policy, changing culture: Steps toward early learning quality improvement in australia." *International Journal of Early Childhood* 43 (2011): 211–25.
25. Eva Cox. "Focus on Working Parents Misses True Value of Universal Early Childhood Services." *The Conversation Online*, 12 May 2015. Available online: http://theconversation.com/focus-on-working-parents-misses-true-value-of-universal-early-childhood-services-41608 (accessed on 11 November 2015).
26. Deborah Brennan, and Rianne Mahon. "State structures and the politics of child care." *Politics & Gender* 7 (2011): 286–93.
27. Liza Griffin. "Where is power in governance? Why geography matters in the theory of governance." *Political Studies Review* 10 (2012): 208–20.
28. Janet Newman. *Modernising Governance New Labour, Policy and Society*. London: Sage, 2001.
29. Helen Dickinson, and Helen Sullivan. "Towards a general theory of collaborative performance: The importance of efficacy and agency." *Public Administration* 92 (2014): 161–77.
30. Andrea Cornwall, and Vera Schatten Coelho. "Spaces for change? The politics of participation in new democratic arenas." In *Spaces for Change? The Politics of Citizen Participation in New Democratic Arenas*. London: Zed Books, 2007, pp. 1–32.
31. Helen Dickinson. *Performing Governance: Partnerships, Culture and New Labour*. London: Palgrave, Macmillan, 2014.
32. Paul Fawcett, and Carsten Daugbjerg. "Explaining governance outcomes: Epistemology, network governance and policy network analysis." *Political Studies Review* 10 (2012): 195–207.
33. Jean-Louis Denis, Ewan Ferlie, and Nicolette Van Gestel. "Understanding hybridity in public organizations." *Public Administration* 93 (2015): 273–89.
34. Roderick Arthur William Rhodes. "Understanding governance: Ten Years on." *Organization Studies* 28 (2007): 1243–64.
35. David Marsh. "The new orthodoxy: The differentiated polity model." *Public Administration* 89 (2011): 32–48.
36. Stephen Bell. "Do we really need a new 'constructivist institutionalism' to explain institutional change?" *British Journal of Political Science* 41 (2011): 883–906.

37. Chris Skelcher, and Helen Sullivan. "Theory-driven approaches to analysing collaborative performance." *Public Management Review* 10 (2008): 751–71.
38. Erik-Hans Klijn, and Chris Skelcher. "Democracy and governance networks: Compatible or not?" *Public Administration* 85 (2007): 587–608.
39. Paul Williams. *Collaboration in Public Policy and Practice: Perspectives on Boundary Spanners*. Bristol: Policy Press, 2012.
40. Chris Skelcher, Helen Sullivan, and Stephen Jeffares. *Hybrid Governance in European Cities: Neighbourhood, Migration and Democracy*. Basingstoke: Palgrave Macmillan, 2013.
41. Shona Hunter. "Ordering differentiation: Reconfiguring governance as relational politics." *Journal of Psycho-Social Studies* 6 (2012): 3–29.
42. Bozeman Barry. "What organization theorists and public policy researchers can learn from one another: Publicness theory as a case-in-point." *Organization Studies* 34 (2013): 169–88.
43. Fredrika Wiesel, and Sven Modell. "From new public management to new public governance? Hybridization and implications for public sector consumerism." *Financial Accountability and Management* 30 (2014): 175–205.
44. Taco Brandsen, Wim van de Donk, and Kim Putters. "Griffins or chameleons? Hybridity as a permanent and inevitable characteristic of the third sector." *International Journal of Public Administration* 28 (2005): 749–65.
45. Tom Christensen, and Per Lægreid. "Complexity and hybrid public administration—Theoretical and empirical challenges." *Public Organization Review* 11 (2010): 407–23.
46. Chris Skelcher, and Steven Rathgeb Smith. "Theorizing hybridity: Institutional logics, complex organizations, and actor identities: The case of nonprofits." *Public Administration* 93 (2015): 433–48. PubMed]
47. Adalbert Evers. "Mixed welfare systems and hybrid organizations: Changes in the governance and provision of social services." *International Journal of Public Administration* 28 (2005): 737–48.
48. Patricia H. Thornton, William Ocasio, and Michael Lounsbury. *The Institutional Logics Perspective: A New Approach to Culture, Structure and Process*. Oxford: Oxford University Press, 2012.
49. Patricia H. Thornton, and William Ocasio. "Institutional logics." In *Handbook of Institutionalism*. Edited by Royston Greenwood, Christine Oliver, Roy Suddaby and Kerstin Sahlin-Andersson. Thousand Oaks: Sage, 2008, pp. 99–129.
50. Roger Friedland, and Robert R. Alford. "Bringing society back in: Symbols, practices and institutional contradictions." In *The New Institutionalism in Organizational Analysis*. Edited by Walter W. Powell and Paul J. DiMaggio. Chicago: University of Chicago Press, 1991, pp. 232–63.
51. Urie Bronfenbrenner. *The Ecology of Human Development: Experiments by Nature and Design*. Cambridge: Harvard University Press, 1979.
52. Oliver E. Williamson. *The Mechanisms of Governance*. Oxford: Oxford University Press, 1996.

53. Chris Skelcher. "What do we mean when we talk abou 'hybrids' and 'hybridity' in public management and governance?" Working Paper, Institute of Local Government Studies, University of Birmingham, Birmingham, UK, 2012. Available online: http://epapers.bham.ac.uk/1601/ (accessed on 3 November 2015).
54. David Mullins, Darinka Czischke, and Gerard van Bortel. "Exploring the meaning of hybridity and social enterprise in housing organisations." *Housing Studies* 27 (2012): 405–17.
55. Brennan Deborah, Cass Bettina, Himmelweit Susan, and Szebehely Marta. "Marketisation of care: Rationales and consequences in Nordic and liberal care regimes." *Journal of European Social Policy* 22 (2012): 377–91.
56. Marianne Fenech, and Jennifer Sumsion. "Promoting high quality early childhood education and care services: Beyond risk management, performative constructions of regulation." *Journal of Early Childhood Research* 5 (2007): 263–83.

In Pursuit of Child and Family Well-Being: Initial Steps to Advocacy

Mary Moeller, Angela McKillip, Ruth Wienk and Kay Cutler

Abstract: Communities across the United States, in both urban and rural areas, are seeking ways to promote well-being for their citizens in sustainable ways. This paper provides a descriptive case study of one rural community that used an inquiry-based approach to ask, "How can we engage our citizens to improve child and family well-being in our community?" The group also wondered "What if Brookings had one place for families to access all family resources that support well-being?" "What if all families had a place where their needs were heard?" and "What if all resources for families looked at the well-being of children and families in a holistic way?" This paper describes the initial journey of a community of practice advocating on several different community levels, including the role of university students, the process of the community of practice formation, its growing connections to community agencies and its initial efforts to build calls to action through participatory research and grassroots community efforts. While conveying a linear narrative, the authors also maintain a focus on the organic processes of knowledge construction and the evolution of a community of practice. Data collection, using the Delphi approach, is underway to access initial ground-up definitions of well-being and to identify areas of focus.

Reprinted from *Soc. Sci.* Cite as: Moeller, M.; McKillip, A.; Wienk, R.; Cutler, K. In Pursuit of Child and Family Well-Being: Initial Steps to Advocacy. *Soc. Sci.* **2016**, 5, 30.

1. Introduction

In announcing a "Year of Inquiry" during the academic year of 2014–2015, the Dean of the College of Education and Human Sciences (EHS) created a call to action that encouraged faculty members to actively explore something that sparked their curiosity. Since several faculty members had expressed curiosity about Reggio-Inspired practices and the work of the Educational Project of Reggio Emilia, Italy, they decided to learn more about that philosophy. In response to this interest and the call to action, Kay Cutler offered to lead a book discussion over the *Hundred Languages of Children: The Reggio Experience in Transformation* [1]. Previously, she and others from the Children's Museum of South Dakota had studied the book, concluding that the book should be read and discussed by a larger cross-section of community residents, including university students, as a provocation. In this way, they meant to stimulate a thought process in Brookings.

The book focuses on the city of Reggio Emilia's educational system; however, the civic community, community members and families are also involved in the governance and leadership of the city-owned schools. In this Italian setting, children are viewed as the city's youngest citizens and as contributing members to their community. In addition, the culture has an embedded, systemic concept of child and family well-being [1]. Often, the published works of Reggio Emilia and nearby cities, such as Pistoia, Italy, focus on the educational components, yet the concept of individual and group well-being is very intricately woven into experiences for young children and families.

The book study offered in the fall of 2014 attracted a cross-section of 15 community/university individuals, including Early Childhood Education faculty members, a Teacher Education faculty member, an Interior Design faculty member, administrators and staff from the Children's Museum of South Dakota, the South Dakota Art Museum Director, a college student, the Dean of the College of EHS, a business entrepreneur and two directors of a local daycare. Using an initial provocation of "Let's consider what we can do here, in Brookings, as we read about the work in Reggio Emilia, Italy", the group met every month and engaged in lively discussions. A chapter written by the mayor of this city at that time sparked a detailed group discussion about the similarities and differences between Reggio Emilia and Brookings. As they read about the organization of the educational office, agency and schools or center through parental representation on the City Education Council, the group's positive energy was palpable. During this particular conversation, they decided to hold a separate meeting outside the regular book study time to capture these newly-recognized thoughts regarding family and child well-being and the process of raising it as a topic for a community-wide conversation.

2. Development of a Community of Practice

This conversation created a turning point with the group transitioning into more than a book study. They recognized their development into a Community of Practice (CoP) with a forming vision and a call to greater action. In terms of the CoP design, they "capture[d] and diffuse[d] existing knowledge to help people improve their practice by providing a forum to identify solutions to common problems and a process to collect and evaluate best practices" ([2], p. 1). CoPs emerge when people come together over a common issue of importance and they develop goals of mutual interest [2]. CoPs can be found in many contexts, such as social, civic, educational and business settings, where groups form to explore topics together [3]. Members might only connect loosely with the CoP at the beginning, but then find that group discussions draw them into deeper involvement [4]. In this case, individuals began researching more broadly into child and family well-being and began bringing their roles and background knowledge into the CoP discussions.

3. Child and Family Well-Being

Child well-being and family well-being can be viewed as two separate constructs, yet family well-being factors often shape the nature of children's well-being factors, and children's well-being factors should be considered in terms of the familial and community context [5–8]. Some familial factors that may influence child well-being include socio-economic status [9,10], parental education levels [11], marital stability [12–14], religious health as measured by participating in religious experiences as a buffer for stress [15–17] and connectedness to a support network [18].

Cultural influences often determine how a group of individuals define well-being, either child or family. For example, the Italian culture views well-being as a group construct defined [19] Donatella Giovanni and measured by context, the environmental stability and relational characteristics [19]. Semanchin Jones, LaLiberte and Piescher find that many models include individual variables focusing on social, physical, cognitive and emotional well-being when looking at child well-being [20,21]. They also find that a few models include contextual, familial aspects or concepts about stability and permanency when coming from a cultural group. Examples include the Relational Worldview Framework created by the National Indian Welfare Association [22] or a more complete viewpoint from the University of Minnesota Center for Spirituality and Healing Model [23]. These two models seem to bring together the being and the context to a greater extent, thus providing a more holistic view of child well-being.

In the Reggio Emilia-inspired practices of Pistoia, Italy, the citizens have engaged in an ongoing dynamic dialogue about what it means to be a child-friendly city. They have created an action plan that involved building places to give children a sense of belonging throughout the city via spaces, signage indicating child-friendly businesses and city policies that ensure more safe urban space for learning and being [24].

Other places around the world have also begun to civically engage in studying children's well-being, such as Melbourne, Australia, as noted in their Kids in Community Report about their city's state of children's well-being [25]. Some cities, also inspired by the work of Reggio Emilia, are working to build capacity to become more civically-engaged communities. For example, Tacoma, Washington, actively seeks to build more opportunities and services on its way to becoming a more child-friendly city [26]. They hosted a one-day conference to ask, "What if children were at the heart of our city?", "What if children came up with community solutions?" and "What if Tacoma were a great place to be a child?" ([26], pp. 5–6). "How would our city look if children helped to solve our community problems? What if families have support and resources before they knew they needed it? What if we did stuff with children instead of for children?" ([27], para. 1).

In pursuing these goals, groups have utilized a variety of methodologies and collected multiple types of data to investigate the status quo and to establish a baseline for improvement. The process of data collection can drive the efforts as citizens seek to understand and to capture the complexities of community. Using multiple measures ensures multiple perspectives, as illustrated in the following list of methodologies from an Australian study that used community surveys, focus groups, stakeholder interviews, service counts, evaluations of access to services, geographical mapping, neighborhood observations, walkability audits and the analysis of census data [25].

After discussing the Melbourne, Australia, report [25] and a local report, the BSC's Benchmarks document [28], the Brookings CoP determined to collect its own data regarding child and family well-being. Maintaining their inquiry-based approach, they also wondered, "How can we civically engage the citizens in our community of Brookings, South Dakota, to dialogue about child and family well-being?" This paper describes how a CoP sought to answer this question. While the journey is by no means complete, the following narrative explains a grassroots process that laid the foundation for ongoing civic engagement.

First, to establish a baseline in Brookings, the CoP began to gather and discuss data from its own community, which put the members in contact with local government and city leaders. One specific study, developed by the Brookings Sustainability Council (BSC) and detailed below in its Benchmarks document, gathered local data to compare Brookings to five "sister" regional cities [28]. As the next step to move the CoP forward and to seek a more official home, the group introduced themselves to the Brookings mayor and requested a meeting.

3.1. Meeting with the Brookings, South Dakota, Mayor

After explaining the origin of the CoP in the book study group, the CoP presented the mayor with a copy of the *Hundred Languages of Children* [1] and gave an overview of its progress to date. They discussed ways the CoP could benefit the city and if it were possible to find a home in the city organizational structure, if the group became more formalized. The mayor encouraged them to review the city policies through the lens of child and family well-being, to identify further data gaps and to ask for time on the BSC's agenda so they would know of this group's existence. He suggested that the BSC would be the best match for this work in the organizational structure of the city.

3.2. Meeting with the Brookings Sustainability Council

Based on the mayor's suggestion, CoP members met with the BSC. At this full council meeting, they briefly described their history, their vision and what they had studied so far, including a discussion of the Brookings Benchmarks document [28]. When the council asked for feedback on the document, the CoP members noted that the earliest educational benchmark occurred when children were 11–12 years old; therefore, no data detailed the earliest years of life and educational quality in the document. The council then requested the group's help in filling in these gaps. When the CoP members asked for the council's feedback, they suggested developing a definition of well-being and creating a vision, mission and framework. The council also suggested that when the CoP had more structure, to establish a connection between the two entities with a member of each group attending the others' meetings.

3.3. Developing an Official Name and Framework for the Advocates for Well-Being

These initial conversations with the mayor and BSC pointed to a clear need to formalize the CoP's organizational structure and to clarify its intentions. Members first developed a strategic framework to aid in identifying who they were, defining well-being and determining action steps (see Figure A1 in Appendix A).

Next, through internal and external audits, they determined an official name for the group, the Advocates for Well-Being (AWB). By selecting the word "Advocate", the group embraced the goal of becoming a voice for others. They intend to speak for or on behalf of others, especially those whose voices are diminished [29]. Inspired by the Reggio-Emilia community, they developed a clear vision for Brookings: a culture that holistically embraces and promotes the well-being of children and families. Their mission: to provide a platform for discussion and engagement by identifying and connecting stakeholders, building advocacy and support for well-being and creating a call to action.

Defining the concept of well-being proved more challenging, yet the AWB had previously embraced guiding principles from their first book study. "Well-being is described as a basic principle guiding the overall sense of community in Reggio Emilia; and one that emerged from a complex-cultural background of history, politics, and economic forces" ([1], p. 37). "The notion of respecting children, more than just loving them, resonated with the group. Respect resembles love in its implicit aim of furtherance, but implies moral relations with others" ([1], pp. 79–80). "In the community of Reggio Emilia, children are viewed as citizens having rights, including civil liability and equal opportunity to a full life. A life of well-being, free of obstacles to holistic development" ([1], p. 84). D. Giovaninni [19] stated the following regarding well-being and children, "Without a basis of well-being, there is no real possibility for growth, for development. This applies to children and families alike. We are talking about well-being in all senses...in relationships...in the environment...in physical requirements. It means for children that their needs are met. Of course, our reflections here about well-being are in the context of a community and are subjective. So, the care and well-being of one person connects to the well-being and care for another." A key word from this vision, holistic, continually guided the

AWB's discussions. For example, the group determined that physical well-being includes the mind, body and spirit.

While the notion of well-being is certainly central to the Reggio-inspired practices, the concept still lacked clearly-defined, culturally-sensitive and measurable components for this context. To build their knowledge base, the AWB turned to the work of Gallup scientists who have been studying the demands of a life well-lived since the mid-20th century. In their research, Gallup conducted a comprehensive global study of 150 countries, providing a lens for over 98% of the world's population. Five distinct factors emerged from this work: career, social, physical, financial and community [30]. The AWB selected this work as a basis for their model and made one important modification: "Children have purpose and intent in their daily activities, but they do not have a "career". In terms of purpose, the wider the range of possibilities for children, the more intense will be their motivations and the richer their experiences" ([1], p. 54). Considering this, the AWB replaced the category of "career" with "inner/self" to describe purpose/intent as a factor of well-being.

The AWB also discussed the term education and its relationship to the five core components at length. They considered if perhaps a sixth component were necessary. Ultimately, the group determined that the concept of education resided within the community as a whole. They concluded that the delicate balance between these core components determines a holistic sense of well-being for a child, and a family. The AWB modified framework then included these descriptors: inner/self, social, physical, financial and community. The descriptors of the core components are intended to clarify and remain fluid as their work continues.

Lastly, determining action steps helped the AWB to also focus on future goals. For example, as the framework developed, they felt a recurring need to add specific detail to the concept of well-being. However, by focusing on the Reggio-inspired practice, the group refrained, believing that further refinement needed to emerge from the community's collective understanding and to be promoted by the community. Still, creating the mission, vision and core components for a guide seemed essential since the community needed to have a better sense of the AWB perspectives as rooted in the book study. Taking this step of describing well-being in general terms was their first action step.

As the second and third action steps, the AWB next identified a need to research their own community to gain perspective and understanding; in a near parallel fashion, implementing the Delphi approach, as described below, contributed to this step. The group also values participatory research to build stakeholder interest in the work and to identify real community needs. Having the community itself periodically refine the concept of well-being and regularly determining areas of need according to a broad range of diverse perspectives, such as a wide variety of representatives from service agencies to family members, themselves, would help identify specific barriers to inclusiveness and access. These perspectives could guide the group in knowing where to advertise or how to ensure under-represented family voices are heard. These action steps would happen in a cyclical fashion through engagement and connection among a broad cross-section of community members. The AWB planned to collectively strategize about action steps or potential solutions, and they envisioned a community summit in the future. The final action step was perhaps the goal from the onset, to impact the community.

3.4. Delphi Approach

One of the challenges at the outset of this project was to broaden the knowledge base of the AWB members. To facilitate this, the AWB prioritized identifying the threats to well-being that were specific to their community. This important step in the advocacy process allowed the AWB to be more deliberate and current in their discussions and plans of action.

Given the scheduling difficulties of gathering community experts and the expense of running a focus group, they chose to implement the Delphi approach to learn about the needs that affect well-being for children and families in Brookings. The Delphi approach, developed by the RAND Corporation and gaining traction in the 1960s, elicits expert opinion on topics via distance. Traditionally, accomplished through mail, this step is now easily completed electronically through the Internet [31]. The Delphi method has the advantage of eliciting expert opinion from a group without the potential for coercive influences that are sometimes observed in committee meetings or focus groups [32].

The AWB implemented the Delphi approach by first identifying local experts in various fields, such as education, healthcare, business, social services, counseling and faith-based institutions. This long process required a considerable amount of brainstorming. Because the experts whose opinions are elicited are the ones who will determine the quality of information, the AWB strategically attempted to identify experts with areas of professional expertise correlated with the well-being framework described earlier in Section 3.3. Finding one person who could address all five of the well-being core components was not the goal of the AWB. Instead, they aimed to compile a panel who could inform all five of the aspects of well-being with their combined knowledge.

Once this group of experts was identified, the AWB began asking questions. The Delphi approach to needs-assessment traditionally asks three rounds of questions [33]. For this study, the first round of questioning simply asked one question: list the top ten indicators of well-being for children and families in the Brookings area. The experts contributed a wide number of responses, identifying more than one hundred seventy initial indicators or potential threats to well-being. These individual indicators were coded using the ATLAS.ti 7 qualitative data analysis software. For the first round of coding, a line-by-line open coding process was utilized. These codes were then analyzed in the software's network view in order to visually organize them in a meaningful manner. The framework of well-being, as the foundation to the AWB work, was utilized as the theory that deductively guided the organization of the codes into a network for further analysis (see Figures A2 and A3). The Figures A2 and A3 analysis showed the trends of three indicators of interest to well-being. The analysis revealed that the AWB intends to further investigate to obtain a clearer picture of the status quo. For example, the access to mental health code tended to be identified as a strong indicator of well-being.

Each AWB member participated in examining the results and contributed to the analysis of the key threats to well-being. After distilling the codes into the top ten indicators necessary for the second round, they contacted the experts again, asking them to rank the indicators in order of importance. Analysis of these data established a consensus of expert opinion, thus eliminating the need for a third round.

Using this Delphi approach to needs assessment, the community experts in Brookings have identified important aspects of well-being for children and families; the top three include access to housing, access to mental health services and access to affordable food. The third indicator from Figures A2 and A3, affordable and nutritious food, surprised the AWB because Brookings is a rural community with rich and productive farmland and is home to a land-grant university with expertise in agricultural research. The apparent lack of access to nutritious food and its high rank as an indicator of concern demonstrates the importance of eliciting information from community experts when conducting a needs analysis. Moreover, this finding illustrates how needs that are fundamental to the well-being of children and family in any area can be invisible to others. However, to verify this understanding of need, the AWB intends to seek out family members' perspectives on well-being, specifically on these three indicators.

3.5. Developing a Call to Action

The AWB's goal to foster community cultural values that embrace and promote the well-being of children and families led to creating a plan for a stakeholder platform discussion. The AWB members asked possible "what if" questions, such as "What if Brookings had one place for families to access all family resources that supported well-being? What if all families had a place where their needs were heard? What if all resources for families worked together to improve well-being, collaborated and supported each other or looked at well-being in a holistic way? Additionally, what if all families in Brookings had a strong and healthy well-being?" in order to develop a framework for the stakeholder platform.

Typically, community agencies attempt to solve education, health and socioeconomic problems for their stakeholders by identifying isolated problems under their jurisdiction based on needs or deficit-based analyses. Once these deficits are determined, separate agencies assume responsibilities for improving conditions in specific areas. Often, the planning process omits the voices of those directly affected by the problem. This isolated approach assumes that the agencies can recognize by themselves what well-being, situated in this context, comprises. Second, the traditional approach assumes that community well-being can be improved by fragmenting and treating the components as independent variables. This simplistic view fails to address the complex interactive nature of communities, wherein education, economics, health and local culture create unique situations. The AWB aims for a holistic approach to community well-being with an inclusive consensus-building model wherein multiple stakeholders, including those directly impacted, collaboratively define a dynamic rather than a static vision of well-being and work together to achieve it.

Initially, the AWB considered three phases of action: raising awareness, educating the community and taking action. They raised awareness by meeting with others during the city's Open Mic Night, a forum to connect with the creative class; and Engage Brookings, a local website with an online tool for gathering community input on city policy. To educate the community and take action, the AWB considered developing a one-day symposium or well-being conference, with follow-up focus groups. For advertising these events, the group recognized that typical media messages may not reach or engage those most directly affected by issues of well-being. The solution required additional, creative ideas for outreach, such as multi-lingual translations for promotional and educational materials, visits over the lunch hour to local manufacturers and transportation services to events.

3.6. Seeking Funding through the Bush Foundation

Creating a call to action requires funding. The AWB applied to the Bush Foundation to seek support for community-wide dialogues on the topic of well-being. Although their application was not funded, the exercise of writing the proposal helped them to clarify their vision and to develop a strategic plan. It included these steps: identify and connect stakeholders, build advocacy and support for well-being and collectively strategize about action steps or potential solutions. Using the Reggio Emilia philosophy, the AWB planned to use "provocations" to attract interest and spark curiosity in community well-being with a focus on their youngest citizens. The AWB continues to seek funding for the call to action.

4. Implications and Future Directions: In Pursuit of Sustainability

The AWB book study generated a shared vision of valuing children as central to community well-being. This main idea serves as the common concern for the CoP that the AWB developed. In reviewing their journey to date, four pieces of work that are common to CoPs and that continue to describe their process emerged. First, their members created relationships through the process of inquiry during the book study; second, they learned from each other and through each other's experiences; third, the AWB coalesced around a common goal that required them to investigate and consider their own community culture; finally, they gained a new understanding of the task before them [2]. However, describing these activities in a linear fashion ignores the cyclical nature of CoP work. For example, the contacts and relationships within and across the community have grown organically as members engage with others. Through collaboration, they enlarged their understanding of community needs that informs new possibilities for actions. Through this increased connectivity, they pursue the goal of a "critical mass needed to evolve into a sustainable entity" ([2], p. 2). Thus, developing a CoP becomes essential for permanent cultural change. Sustainability in this context means a community that embraces the well-being of children and families as its core institutional value and seeks continual renewal of that vision.

4.1. Continued Data Collection

The Delphi method is limited because it only provides an outsider's etic perspective of the needs of the target population. While the experts, in many cases, work closely with the at-risk and in-need population of the city, they are not living in those conditions themselves. This naturally imposes a limit to the scope of information, as well as a contextualized understanding of the possible threats to the well-being of children and families. To address this information deficit, the AWB are considering a participatory method of information gathering that produces a more inclusive dataset.

In addition, utilizing participatory methodology, such as Photo Voice, has the capacity to empower the at-risk population [34]. From a Freirean context, this benefit addresses the weakness of the Delphi in that a participatory approach does not treat the target population as objects of research. Instead, marginalized people are recognized as the experts on their own well-being with voices that have equal weight in the needs-assessment process [35]. This type of community empowerment and coming to voice is highly consistent with the goals and vision of the AWB. Using an approach to knowledge gathering from adults also aligns ideologically with a community-initiated approach to knowledge building that is central to the Reggio Emilia teaching philosophy. All of these ideals provided the impetus for the Brookings AWB. In their recent meeting, they reviewed survey data from local agency employees who work with children and families. Since families have not yet been asked directly about child and family well-being, this will be their next step in data collection in order to gather many perspectives and further refine the data.

4.2. Deeper Connections with Community

The AWB has sought to create deeper connections with area agencies, such as Brookings *Area United Way*. Last fall, the AWB met with the Executive Director to explore ways to connect with existing initiatives. Connecting to those and creating an integrated call to action are the strategic goal. The AWB also met with the *Brookings Economic Development Corporation* Entrepreneurship Program Coordinator to discuss possible connections to their BEDC Visioning Charettes and strategic planning document. The AWB identified two ways to assist with the BEDC's strategic goals: (1) to engage the university personnel in meaningful partnerships; and (2) to create an engaging social ecosystem in the communities with access for all residents. Through dialogue, the AWB decided to focus primarily on influencing this last goal. The AWB also have been invited to circle back around and meet a second time with the Brookings Sustainability Council after a second Open Mic conversation.

Recognizing Undergraduates as an Asset: Several members of the original book study group have university faculty appointments in teacher education. As such, they occasionally mentor students majoring in education or a related area, who seek opportunities to dig deeper, to serve children in extended ways or to research issues related to teaching. Some of these university students also look for opportunities to "honor" a course to fulfill requirements for the Honors College; they look for undergraduate research opportunities, and the university encourages this activity as a way to enrich student experiences; advocacy is one of those experiences.

Including undergraduates as AWB members also benefits the group because students add energy and creative perspectives. In addition, students bring possible collaborative opportunities that extend the group's reach and provide resources. For example, currently, a university student who is also a member of the Student Program of the National Education Association, an organization that offers grants to promote collaboration and outreach between university students and the community, wrote a proposal to fund the AWB's work. This proposal supported an educational goal for the community because the AWB can now establish a small library of materials and books related to well-being. Undergraduate research and data collection possibilities also exist within this work, as either research assistants or full partnership collaborations.

4.3. Selection of a New Text

To keep the AWB members engaged in their own learning, they have selected *A More Beautiful Question: The Power of Inquiry to Spark Breakthrough Ideas*, by Warren Berger [36], for their next collaborative book study. Continuing with a book discussion allows them to reach out to community members, build the CoP and widen the circle of AWB. Since their first book study, six key community members have joined the core group as active members. This process epitomizes the cyclic nature of inquiry and CoP development.

4.4. Alternative Approaches to the Call to Action

Pursuing the AWB's goals requires finding new funding sources, seeking support from foundations and finding or creating a home within the existing institutional and community structures in a way that is transparent, supportive and effective. These are the challenges that the AWB faces.

The opportunity to capture their work by writing this current manuscript in the group's development adds perspective in a similar way that writing and reviewing the work accomplished in the grant writing process. The AWB find themselves immersed in the CoP life cycle as they move through the different phases of growth, knowledge generation and revitalization [3].

5. Conclusions

Their decision to pursue a cultural transformation by building a more sustainable, approachable, family-friendly community has made AWB aware of the many organizations working to realize these very same goals. The AWB will continue to study and benefit from the strategies, methods and findings emerging from other locations. A second lesson learned is that a grassroots effort takes times and a financial commitment in order for the call to action to move forward. In addition, the second step of the call to action, the educational outreach, requires money and expertise. A third lesson learned is that this process occurs in cycles similar to that of a CoP. The envisioning process that was part of the book study discussion energized their group. They coalesced around the possibilities for their community, and even more they began to wonder what Brookings might look like as a model community. As they work on launching the next cycle, the AWB members wonder how to go about achieving a larger goal to impact the region and even the state. Those thoughts motivate and shape their work: to foster a community culture that values family and child well-being in this city.

Author Contributions: Kay Cutler and others conceived of the idea of the book study. Angela McKillip and Kate Treiber designed the Advocates of Well-Being framework. Ruth Wienk and others designed the survey study and collected the data. Ruth Wienk analyzed the data. Mary Moeller, Angela McKillip, Kay Cutler and Kate Treiber wrote the grant proposal. Others in the Advocates for Well-Being group developed the call to action. All authors wrote the paper.

Conflicts of Interest: The authors declare no conflict of interest.

Abbreviations

The following abbreviations are used in this manuscript:

AWB	Advocates for Well-Being
BEDC	Brookings Economic Development Corporation
BSC	Brookings Sustainability Council
CoP	Community of Practice
EHS	College of Education and Human Sciences
RAND	Rand Corporation; RAND was developed from the terms Research and Development, yet has been called Rand as an established name
TEDx	A Technology, Entertainment and Design event that is independently organized, not sponsored by the TED nonprofit

Appendix A.

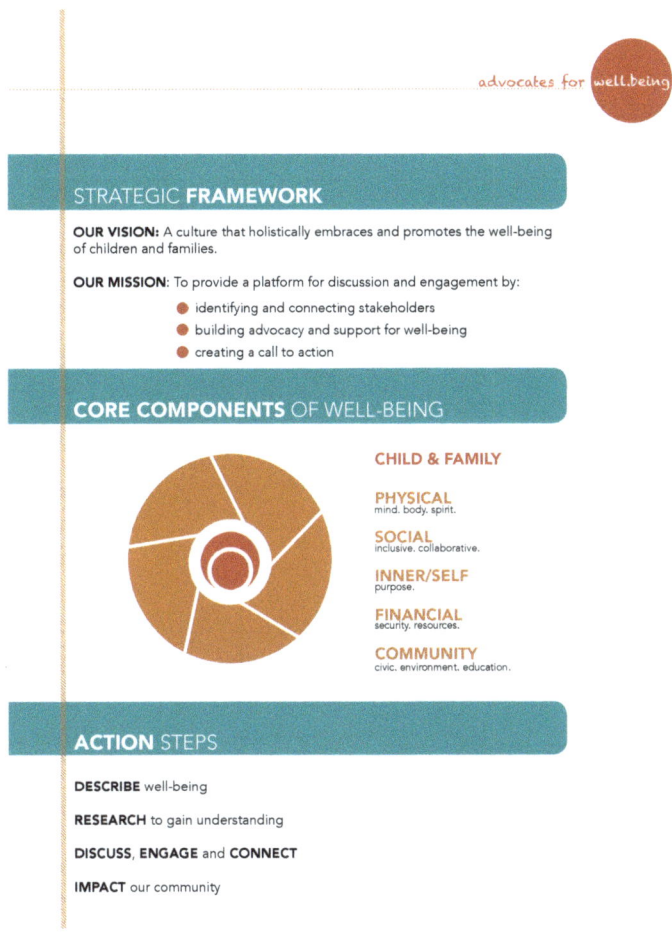

Figure A1. Advocates for Well-Being Framework with descriptors of the components of child and family well-being.

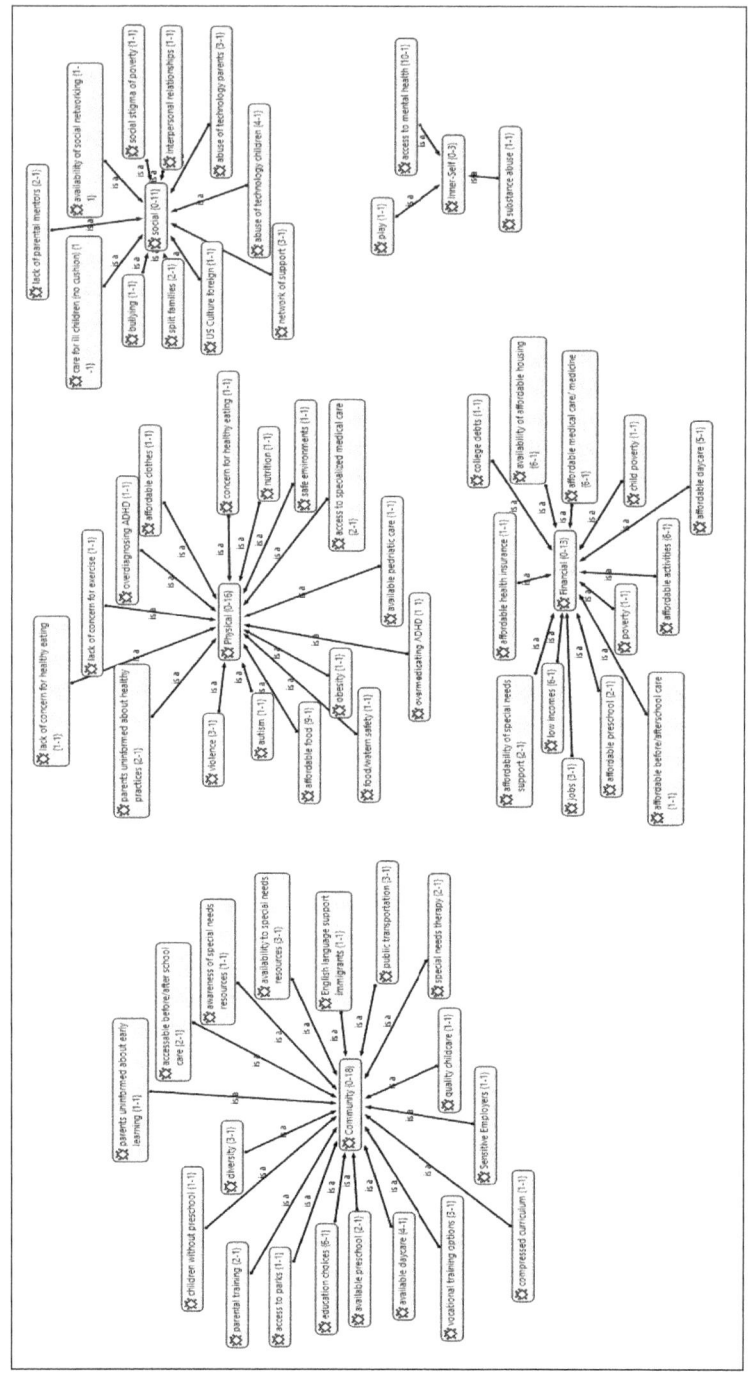

Figure A2. Identified Threats to Well-Being.

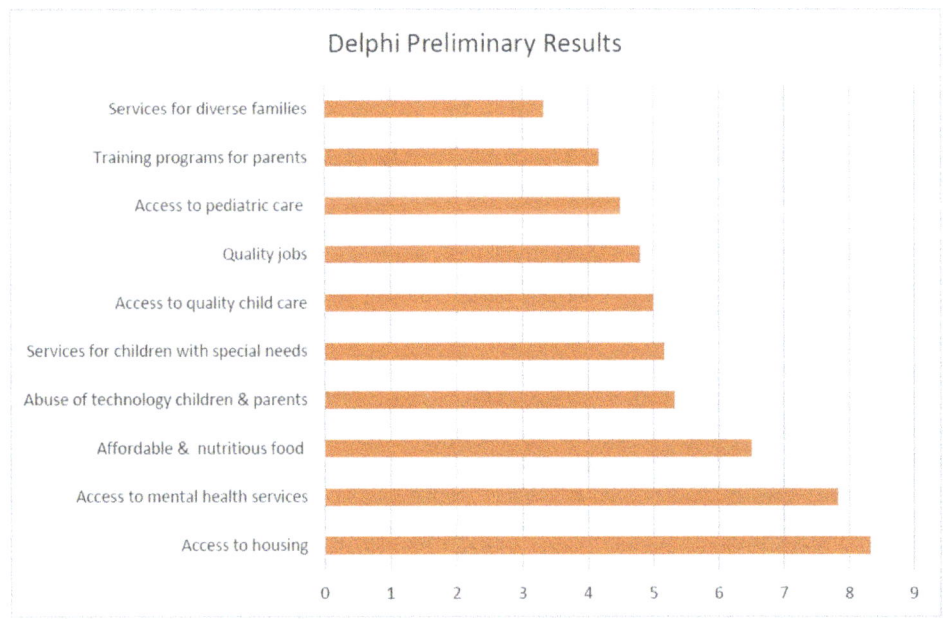

Figure A3. Delphi preliminary results.

References

1. Edwards, Carolyn, Lella Gandini, and George Forman. *Hundred Languages of Children: The Reggio Experience in Transformation*, 3rd ed. Santa Barbara: Praeger, 2012.
2. Cambridge, Darren, Soren Kaplan, and Vicki Suter. "Community of practice design guide: A step by step guide for designing and cultivating communities of practice in higher education." 2015. Available online: http://net.educause.edu/ir/library/pdf/NLI0531.pdf (accessed on 30 April 2015).
3. Wenger, Etienne. "Communities of practice. Learning as a social system." *Systems Thinker* 9 (1998): 2–3.
4. Lave, Jean, and Etienne Wenger. *Situated Learning. Legitimate Peripheral Participation*. Cambridge: University of Cambridge Press, 1991.
5. Gosselin, Julie, Lyzon Babchishin, and Elisa Romano. "Family transitions and children's well-being during adolescence." *Journal of Divorce & Remarriage* 56 (2015): 569–89.
6. Luthar, Suniya, and Lucia Ciciolla. "Who mothers mommy? Factors that contribute to mothers' well-being." *Developmental Psychology* 51 (2015): 1812–23.
7. Coleman, James S. "Social capital in the creation of human capital." *American Journal of Sociology* 94 (1988): S95–120.
8. Bronfenbrennor, Urie. *The Ecology of Human Development: Experiments by Nature and Design*. Cambridge: Harvard University Press, 1979.

9. Conger, Rand D., and M. Brent Donnellan. "An interactionist perspective on the socioeconomic context of human development." *Annual Review of Psychology* 58 (2007): 175–99.
10. McLoyd, Vonnie C., Toby Epstein Jayaratne, Rosario Ceballo, and Julio Borquez. "Unemployment and work interruption among African American single mothers: Effects on parenting and adolescent socioemotional functioning." *Child Development* 65 (1994): 562–89.
11. Ramey, Garey, and Valerie A. Ramey. "The rug rat race." In *Brookings Papers on Economic Activity Economic Studies Program*. Washington: The Brookings Institution, 2010, pp. 129–99.
12. Brown, Susan L., Wendy D. Manning, and Krista K. Payne. "Family structure and children's economic well-being: Incorporating same-sex cohabiting mother families." *Population Research and Policy Review* 35 (2016): 1–21.
13. McLanahan, Sara, and Isabel Sawhill. "Marriage and child wellbeing revisited: Introducing the issue." *Future of Children* 25 (2015): 3–9.
14. Ribar, David. "Why marriage matters for child well-being." *The Future of Children* 15 (2005): 11–27.
15. Wen, Ming. "Parental participation in religious services and parent and child well-being: Findings from the National Survey of Americas Families." *Journal of Religious Health* 53 (2014): 1539–61.
16. Garcia, Gloria, Christopher G. Ellison, Thankam S. Sunil, and Terrence D. Hill. "Religion and selected health behaviors among Latinos in Texas." *Journal of Religion and Health* 52 (2013): 18–31.
17. Levin, Jeff. "'And let us make us a name': Reflections on the future of the religion and health field." *Journal of Religion and Health* 48 (2009): 125–45.
18. Amato, Paul R. "The Impact of family formation change on the cognitive, social and emotional well-being of the next generation." *The Future of Children* 15 (2005): 75–96.
19. Giovaninni, Donatella (Pedagogista of the Preschools, Pistoia, Italy). Personal communication, 22 February 2012.
20. Serbati, Sara, Monica Pivetti, and Gianmaria Gioga. "Child Well-Being Scales (CWBS) in the assessment of children and families in home care intervention: An empirical study." *Child and Family Social Work* 20 (2013): 446–58.
21. Jones, Semanchin, LaLiberte Traci Annette, and Kristine Piescher. "Defining and strengthening child well-being in child protection." *Children and Youth Services Review* 54 (2015): 57–70.
22. Cross, Terry. *The Relational Worldview and Child Well-Being. CW 360: Attending to Well-Being in Child Welfare*. St. Paul: Center for Advanced Studies in Child Welfare, School of Social Work, University of Minnesota, 2014.
23. Center for Spirituality & Healing. "The Wellbeing Model." 2013. Available online: http://www.takingcharge.csh.umn.edu/wellbeing-model (accessed on 10 March 2016).
24. Rauch, Andrea. *L'immagianrio Bambini: The Educational Experiences of Pistoia City Council in the Drawing and Graphics*. Florence: Edizioni Junior, 2003.

25. Goldfeld, Sharon, Talya Mathews, Sally Brinkman, G. Woolcock, Jenny Myers, Paul Kershaw, Ilan Katz, Rob Tanton, and J. Wiseman. *The Kids in Communities Study: Measuring Community Level Factors Influencing Children's Development*. Melbourne: Murdoch Childrens Research Institute, 2010.
26. Children's Museum of Tacoma. "A Symposium on Our Youngest Citizens: Childhood as a Community Value." 23 September 2014. Available online: https://www.playtacoma.org/symposium (accessed on 11 September 2015).
27. Thrive Washington. "Hundreds Gather in Tacoma to Explore What it Means to Build a Child-Centered Community." Available online: https://thrivewa.org/hundreds-gather-tacoma-explore-means-build-child-centered-community/ (accessed on 10 February 2016).
28. Brookings Sustainability Council. *Brookings Benchmarks Baseline Sustainability Report*. Edited by Kate Hillfill. Brookings: Brookings Sustainability Council, 2014.
29. Maurer, Trent. "Giving Voice to SoTL." Paper presented at the SoTL Commons Conference, Savannah, GA, USA, 30 March 2016.
30. Rath, Tom, and Jim Harter. *Wellbeing: The Five Essential Elements*. New York: Gallup Press, 2010.
31. Gordon, Theodore Jay. "The delphi method." *Futures Research Methodology* 3 (1994): 1–29.
32. Brown, Bernice B. *Delphi Process: A Methodology Used for the Elicitation of Opinions of Experts (No. RAND-P-3925)*. Santa Monica: RAND Corp., 1968.
33. Hsu, Chia-Chen, and Brian A. Sandford. "The Delphi technique: Making sense of consensus." *Practical Assessment Research & Evaluation* 12 (2007): 1–8.
34. Strack, Robert W., Cathleen Magill, and Kara McDonagh. "Engaging youth through photovoice." *Health Promotion Practice* 5 (2004): 49–58.
35. Freire, Pablo. *Education for Critical Consciousness*. London: Bloomsbury Publishing, 1973, vol. 1.
36. Berger, Warren. *A More Beautiful Question: The Power of Inquiry to Spark Breakthrough Ideas*. New York: Bloomsbury USA, 2014.

Community Engaged Leadership to Advance Health Equity and Build Healthier Communities

Kisha Holden, Tabia Akintobi, Jammie Hopkins, Allyson Belton, Brian McGregor, Starla Blanks and Glenda Wrenn

Abstract: Health is a human right. Equity in health implies that ideally everyone should have a fair opportunity to attain their full health potential and, more pragmatically, that no one should be disadvantaged from achieving this potential. Addressing the multi-faceted health needs of ethnically and culturally diverse individuals in the United States is a complex issue that requires inventive strategies to reduce risk factors and buttress protective factors to promote greater well-being among individuals, families, and communities. With growing diversity concerning various ethnicities and nationalities; and with significant changes in the constellation of multiple of risk factors that can influence health outcomes, it is imperative that we delineate strategic efforts that encourage better access to primary care, focused community-based programs, multi-disciplinary clinical and translational research methodologies, and health policy advocacy initiatives that may improve individuals' longevity and quality of life.

Reprinted from *Soc. Sci.* Cite as: Holden, K.; Akintobi, T.; Hopkins, J.; Belton, A.; McGregor, B.; Blanks, S.; Wrenn, G. Community Engaged Leadership to Advance Health Equity and Build Healthier Communities. *Soc. Sci.* **2016**, *5*, 2.

---

1. Health Disparities: A Global Challenge

A recent report of the World Health Organization entitled *U.S. Health in International Perspective: Shorter Lives, Poorer Health* documented the alarming implications of poor health status among many individuals, families, and communities [1]. This landmark report helps to delineate from a global perspective, comparisons among seventeen peer countries relative to the issue of life expectancy, selected medical conditions, and health outcomes particularly concerning infant mortality and low birth weight, injuries and homicides, disability, adolescent pregnancy and sexually transmitted infections, HIV and AIDS, drug-related deaths, obesity and diabetes, heart disease, mental health, and chronic lung disease. One notable and consistent finding suggested that individuals that are most negatively impacted, suffer the greatest, and highest at-risk for deleterious outcomes represent poor, underserved, and vulnerable communities inundated by individuals that live in poverty. These harsh realities warrant further examination and the critical need to determine the role of public health in the quest for global health equity.

Equity in health implies that ideally everyone should have a fair opportunity to attain their full health potential and, more pragmatically, that no one should be disadvantaged from achieving this potential [2,3]. In many nations, social justice, environmental, and economic issues may impact an individual's livelihood, exposure to illness, and risk of early mortality according to a 2008 report of the World Health Organization's Commission on Social Determinants of Health (CSDH) [4]. When extreme differences in health are significantly associated with social disadvantages, the differences can be labeled as health inequities; and in most cases these differences are: (1) systematic and avoidable; (2) facilitated and exacerbated by circumstances in which people live, work, and contend will illness; and (3) may be intensified by political, economic, and/or social influences [4]. Even in countries such as the U.S. that have economic power and several individuals with adequate resources, persons belonging to lower socioeconomic levels experience the worst health outcomes [4].

It is imperative that public health professionals, researchers, clinicians and policy makers embrace lead roles to bridge the gap between the rich and the poor concerning health issues, by promoting health equity and setting guidelines for global health initiatives. In order to address the plight of health inequities, social justice must be expanded to reach people on a larger scale which is more inclusive and less exclusive. We need leaders that will actively promote the CSDH three principles of action: (1) enhance daily living conditions in which people are born, grow, live, work, and age; (2) address inequitable distribution of power, money, and resources; and (3) accurately measure the issues, assess action plans, increase the knowledge base, create a workforce of persons trained in social determinants of health, and increase awareness about social determinants of health [5]. Moreover, one of the overarching goals for Healthy People 2020 is to "achieve health equity, eliminate disparities, and improve the health of all groups". This can be accomplished with ethical and focused public health leaders at the helm. Using the public health approach which starts and ends with surveillance, indicates that it is appropriate to: (1) accurately define the health problem or opportunity; (2) determine the cause or risk factors involved; (3) determine what works to prevent or ameliorate the problem; and (4) determine how to replicate the strategy more broadly and evaluate the impact [5].

Addressing the multi-faceted health needs of ethnically and culturally diverse individuals in the United States is a complex issue that requires inventive strategies to reduce risk factors and buttress protective factors to promote greater well-being among individuals, families, and communities. There is growing diversity of various ethnicities and nationalities. There are significant changes in the constellation of multiple risk factors that can influence health outcomes, and it is imperative that we delineate strategic efforts that encourage better access to primary care, focused community-based programs, multi-disciplinary clinical and translational research methodologies, and health policy advocacy initiatives that may improve individuals' longevity and quality of life. These issues have particular relevance for vulnerable and underserved populations, including African Americans, which have lower life expectancies compared to Caucasians in the U.S. [6].

2. Addressing Health Disparities from a Community Perspective

Community design assumes a major role in the overall health outcomes of community members. The built environment is defined as the "settings designed, created, modified, and maintained by human efforts, such as homes, schools, workplaces, neighborhoods, parks, roadways, and transit systems" [7]. Designs in the built environment, as well as natural landscapes, affect body structure and internal health as food environment and physical activity can be abundant or limited within one's built environment. Design may affect accessibility to healthy drinking water or good quality air for breathing. Where one lives forms the basis for his/her health outcomes. It can enhance our quality of life, or it can adversely affect our very well-being. If a neighborhood lacks fundamental components within the built environment to support sufficient employment and education, access to healthy food options, sustainable active living space, and access to quality health care, then the risk of suffering from one or more chronic conditions exponentially increases for its residents [8].

Despite decades of research and programmatic enterprises, chronic medical conditions (such as diabetes and cardiovascular disease) remain a significant public health problem in the United States, especially for low income, racial and ethnic minority communities [9]. A myriad of social, structural, psychosocial, and environmental factors, including poor access to health care, food insecurity and lack of access to affordable healthy foods, lack of physical activity, and compromised mental and behavioral health, impact community members' ability to participate in overall health-promoting behaviors, thereby exacerbating health outcomes [10]. Public health efforts to accelerate chronic disease prevention and reduce health inequities are increasingly focused on policy, systems, and environmental (PSE) approaches. Leading organizations such as the Centers for Disease Control and Prevention (CDC), Institutes of Medicine (IOM), the Robert Wood Johnson Foundation (RWJF), and the National Institutes of Health (NIH) have called for increased efforts at the state and local levels to advance such approaches. Changing policies and environments to promote active living and healthy eating require cooperation among diverse sectors [11]. Moreover, the CDC has highlighted the importance of coordination among multiple sectors as a key to successful efforts [12]. The IOM has emphasized the importance of engaging the non-health sectors in changing policies and environments to address chronic disease [13]. Collaboration should involve people or organizations from multiple sectors (e.g., planners, developers, media specialists, neighborhood residents, elected officials) and geographical strata (e.g., state, regional, local, neighborhood) [12]. Collaborative groups that promote stakeholder engagement and interaction have been associated with increased relevance, feasibility, and long-term sustainability of initiatives [14]. These groups have the potential to develop and maintain strategies to increase opportunities by leveraging resources, sharing knowledge, and building relationships [13]. The collaborative effort reflected in this proposal reflects a commitment to PSE approaches and the engagement of key stakeholders across sectors.

There are persistent gaps in many underserved, at-risk, and vulnerable communities for health promotion and disease prevention [15,16]. Social, emotional, and mental (SEM) problems can negatively impact an individual's lifestyle behaviors that may increase their risk for a myriad of chronic disease [17]. One must consider the dynamic direct, indirect, and bi-directional relationships between SEM wellness and lifestyle behaviors such as physical activity [18], healthy eating [19], and tobacco-free living [20,21]. In particular, symptoms of a mental disorder, exposure to stressors, lack of social support, and the degree to which they believe behavior change is possible (self-efficacy) may harmfully impact: (1) receptivity to engaging in healthy lifestyle behaviors; (2) initiating behavior change; (3) resiliency when faced with setbacks and challenges; and (4) sustaining behavior changes on a long-term basis.

As health care reform is implemented, there is an opportunity to improve community health and health care. The crucial next step in advancing our scientific knowledge within selected populations is to establish multidimensional strategies that include communities, clinic systems, and community consumers' collaboration that may bolster the potential for successes in the reduction of health disparities among vulnerable populations, including many African Americans. Specifically, part of the solution entails utilizing community based participatory approaches that: (1) leverage the experience and influence of community stakeholders to promote policy, environmental, and systems advocacy; (2) advance approaches for comprehensive integrated systems of care; and (3) improve community health leadership competencies and skills. Public health has an integral role in reducing health inequity, particularly concerning the distribution of resources through health education, creating a workforce of persons that target underserved communities, and increasing awareness about social determinants of health among bourgeoning professionals.

3. Community Engaged Approaches to Build Healthier Communities

3.1. Understanding Community Based Participatory Approaches

Historically, academic research in communities existed in which the academic institution received significant benefit; however, the community held no control of research projects and tended not to receive any benefit. Community-based participatory research (CBPR) is a research approach that emphasizes community-academic partnership and shared leadership in the planning, implementation, evaluation and dissemination of initiatives. Among the advantages of CBPR are strengthened neighborhood-campus relationships, improved research question relevance, enhanced research recruitment, implementation, collective dissemination, and mutual benefit for a diverse group of stakeholders [22–27].

The evolution and application of community based participatory research (CBPR) in communities has led to increased research participation and community ownership, globally. Conceptually, it is anticipated that through utilizing CBPR, outcomes will include not only answering a research question and reaping associated benefits, but also addressing community-identified social, economic or policy priorities [25]. One of the tenets of CBPR is the principle that researchers who want to conduct effective health research must invest time and resources in building partnerships with community-based organizations or neighborhood residents who are gatekeepers to establishing and maintaining community buy-in, ownership and sustainability. Ideally, community residents are equal or senior partners throughout the research process [26].

Previous meta-analyses and reviews have been conducted to understand CBPR, provide practical recommendations in its utilization, and to evaluate its research value, impact on health status and systems change [28]. Jagosh *et al.* [22] identifies contextual determinants of CBPR success that include the ability to collaboratively navigate conflict, negotiate and build consensus [29]. Among the results of successful partnerships are culturally and contextually tailored research, enhanced participant recruitment, and project sustainability. A recent meta-analysis of CBPR initiatives utilizing 46 instruments identified empowerment and community capacity measures among primary CBPR outcomes [30].

3.2. Benefits of Establishing a Community Coalition Board and Engagement to Build Healthier Communities

Establishing a governing body that ensures community-engaged research is challenging when: (1) academicians have not previously been guided by neighborhood experts in the evolution of a community's ecology; (2) community members have not led discussions regarding their health priorities; or (3) academic and neighborhood experts have not historically worked together as a single body with established rules to guide roles and operations [31,32]. In the context of CBPR a community coalition board (CCB), composed of local stakeholders who serve and reside in prioritized communities adds substance to research and other health initiatives by providing local leadership and guidance on the most appropriate positioning of interventions, modes of community engagement for data collection, and access to neighborhood residents and leaders critical to effective public health initiatives [33,34]. Further, community residents' lived experience as a group that may have experienced exploitation in research all the more requires that they not only hold a place at the research development and implementation table, but that their recommendations translate to action. Ideally, community residents should be equal or senior partners in relation to academic stakeholders on such boards, informing the development of the evaluation question, logic model, appropriate recruitment and retention strategies, and, most importantly, the translation of results to inform decision making, policy change, or subsequent research [33].

The Morehouse School of Medicine Prevention Research Center (PRC) was based on the applied definition of CBPR, in which research is conducted with, not on, communities in a partnering relationship faced with high levels of poverty, a lack of neighborhood resources, a plague of chronic diseases, and basic distrust in the research process as metropolitan Atlanta community members initially expressed their apprehension about participating in yet another partnership with an academic institution to conduct what they perceived as meaningless research in their neighborhoods. At the outset, the PRC created a governance model in which the community would serve as the "senior partner" in its relationship with the medical school and other academic and agency collaborators. The PRC is governed by a Community Coalition Board (CCB), to which all the identified partners belong, but community representatives hold the preponderance of power, literally putting them at the forefront of all CBPR and related approaches. Board members, including academic, agency, and neighborhood representatives, truly represent the community and its priorities. Academic representatives include the faculty and staff that are frequently engaged in carrying out the research service or training initiatives affiliated with the PRC. Agency staff (e.g., health department staff, school board representative) may not live in the community where they work, but their agencies serve the communities. Their input has value, but represents the goals and objectives of their organization, rather than the lived experience of a resident. Residents of the community—"neighborhood representatives"—are in the majority, and one always serves as Board Chair, as opposed to agency or academic members of the CCB. The PRC's CCB serves as a policy-making board—not an "advisory board", which has created an opportunity for community partners to have an active voice in directing the operations of and sustainability for the Center.

Central to establishing such a board was an iterative process of disagreement, dialogue, and compromise that ultimately resulted in the identification of what academicians needed from neighborhood board members and what they, in turn, would offer communities Not unlike other new social exchanges, each partner had to first learn, respect, and then value what the other considers a worthy benefit in return for participating on the board [35,36]. According to a former PRC CCB chair, community members allow researchers conditional access to their communities to engage in research with an established community benefit. Benefits to CCB members include the research findings as well as education, the building of skills and capacity, and an increased ability to access and navigate clinical and social services [36–41]. Benefits to board members in similar partnerships may also include dissemination of relevant and actionable research findings, the building of skills and capacity, and an increased ability to access and navigate clinical and social services. Among benefits to academic researchers are established community trust and relationships with partners beyond the community who have direct relation with the resources and partners that serve as local strengths and resources towards addressing health and social disparities and advancing health equity.

Critical to maintaining a community driven governance board are established bylaws that provide a blue-print for the governing body As much as possible, board members should be people who truly represent the community and its priorities. The differing values of academic and community CCB representatives are acknowledged and coexist within an established infrastructure that supports collective functioning to address community health promotion initiatives [33,42]. Lessons learned in CBPR community coalition board development and sustainability are detailed below:

- Engagement in effective community coalition boards is developed through multi-directional learning of each partner's values and needs [38]
- Community coalition boards are built and sustained over time to ensure community ownership through established rules and governance structures
- Trust and relationship building are both central to having neighborhood and research experts work together to shape community-engaged research agendas
- Maintaining a community coalition board requires ongoing communication and feedback, beyond formal monthly or quarterly meetings, to keep members engaged

3.3. Strengthening Community-Academic Partnerships

To support building healthier communities, it is imperative to have community-academic partnerships which can garner a mutually beneficial experience. In the book, *Building Health Coalitions in the Black Community* [43], some of the building blocks of a strong partnerships include: clear identification of an issue/concern/topic, gaining support of key gatekeepers, stakeholders and agencies, establishing guiding principles including decision-making and action teams or committees, consensus building about the work to be accomplished, mapping of assets to enhance working relationships, effective communication and sharing of information, and performing continuous quality improvement/process evaluation of activities. Moreover, some of the characteristics of successful community-academic partnerships include:

- Attention to the fundamental tasks of long range planning, recruitment of members, and inter- and intra-coalition communication
- Monitoring of legislative and fiscal changes affecting the coalition and its members
- Leadership that emphasizes both task-oriented and interpersonal functions of the group
- Management of conflict within the coalition while maintaining its presence in the community
- Model whereby all members experience a sense of ownership and that they have impacted the action plan and implementation
- Diverse socialization opportunities (e.g., retreats, in-service training, workshops, *etc.*)
- Mentoring and training that focuses on developing leadership skills for members
- Aggressive fundraising and appropriate resource allocation

It is vital that both community members and academic institutions are mutually respected to avoid common reasons for coalitions and partnerships to fail, which include:

- Sabotage
- Interpersonal conflict and long standing feuds between partnering organizations
- Lack of genuine inclusion
- Hidden agendas of coalition members that can negatively influence other individuals
- Lack of group ownership
- Poor information/communication flow
- Lack of cultural competence
- Poor leadership

4. Significance of Ethical Leadership in Promoting Community Health

In the Institute of Medicine's landmark report, *The Future of Public Health* [44] one major issue promoted was "the need for leaders is too great to leave their emergence to chance". Moreover, we contend that principles espoused in the book, *Ethical Leadership: The Quest for Character, Civility and Community* [45] are essential to progressive innovative approaches and initiatives to build healthier communities. It is critical that leaders adopt leadership principles inclusive of: (1) insight—the importance of self-awareness, personal biases, and having empathy for others circumstances; (2) integrity—ethical governance and developing congruence between one's own values and one's actions; (3) synergy—learning the ability to work cooperatively and effectively with others in ways that empower individuals to use their gifts and make contributions that can benefit all parties; (4) sharing the "commitment to action"—developing the motivation to translate knowledge into action, foster buy-in and support, and to become actively involved in individual and collaborative efforts to foster personal and social change; and (5) impact—promoting positive civic engagement and social responsibility through an ethic of service and a concern for justice. In part, it will require focused training in these domains for community leaders to advance health equity. Examples of model leadership development programs are within the Satcher Health Leadership Institute (SHLI) at Morehouse School of Medicine (MSM). For example, SHLI's Community Health Leadership Program, Health Policy Leadership Fellowship, Integrated Care Leadership Program, and Smart and Secure Parent Leadership Development Program have established pioneering strategies for preparing diverse community members, post-doctoral health professionals, physician leaders, and parents for tackling the myriad of complex and intricate health issues that plague underserved vulnerable communities.

Effective and ethical leadership is a critical key to success in the quest for building healthier communities. According to a first-ever study of U.S. medical schools in the area of social mission, MSM ranks #1 in the nation [46]. In order to encourage community health and ethical responsibility for future health care providers, researchers, and public health professional priority regarding leadership training is critical. There is leadership capacity in all of us; and we must help to develop that capacity because leadership matters. Leaders must be good learners, continually learning more about themselves, those they lead, and the cause or missions for which they work. Focused initiatives and cross-cultural collaborations will be achieved as we continue to transform the science of ethical decision-making and discovery in research, health promotion, and practice. U.S. based public health professionals, practitioners, research scientists, policymakers, community leaders, and individual consumers collectively have unique roles as thought leaders in the design, implementation, and evaluation of innovative strategies to promote community health and advance health equity.

5. Understanding Cultural Values and Implications of Planned Community-Based Activities

While socioeconomic, physical, and social environments can affect opportunities for healthy behaviors, the culture of communities must also be taken into account when developing interventions and seeking to engage communities for change. Research on health and health disparities demonstrate the importance of the built environment and the impact that systemic and structural changes can provide in relation to impacting health equality [47]; however the role of culture in engaging communities, designing interventions and implementation cannot be overlooked.

For example, an urban African American experience often lacks representation and input into community planning and infrastructure development as well as a lack of perceived power in engaging in decision-making about resource allocation. Discriminatory policies and practices tied to race/ethnicity and socioeconomic status have resulted in disinvestment in urban African American communities and resulted in underrepresented and disenfranchised residents [48]. Understanding the challenges and lack of engagement of urban communities in conjunction with the cultural mistrust is a critical but often overlooked aspect of research and intervention design. Research shows that when residents take an active role in improving neighborhood conditions, a positive effect on health results [49]. However, positioning health education as a permanent function requires the infrastructure for reliable and culturally congruent programming [50] that accounts for community input, non-traditional power centers, faith-based leaders and engagement of traditionally underrepresented segments of the community. Acknowledging the role of racism in health inequities and committing to addressing the root causes of health inequities is essential for establishing trust with community groups and in the development of successful culturally competent programming.

Despite the importance of addressing culture in community level interventions designed to improve health by addressing policies, systems, and the environment, there is a dearth of research focusing on culture and the built environment. Programs such as the Philadelphia Mural Arts Program [51] and Project ACHIEVE [50,52] are examples of community-engaged efforts that facilitate cultural tailoring of interventions to impact the physical environment and policy respectively. While there are many programs that operate within a community-engaged framework addressing population health, a gap remains in identifying best practices in attending to culture up front when designing place-based interventions [53].

Moreover, significant consideration that should be more supported in public health and a top priority of health delivery management teams is cultural competency training and education. According to the U.S. Census Bureau, non-Hispanic whites will comprise the numerical minority by 2050; and diversification is imperative for health care organizations to be more equipped to address cultural issues of varied patient populations that are served [54]. Cultural competence rests on a continuum and requires providers and public health professionals to reflect on their own identity, biases, and belief systems; and it is important to respect, understand, and accept other cultures [55].

In conclusion, to achieve the goal of lasting environmental change in the context of diverse communities, it is critical to: (1) engage neighborhood residents from the outset to build social capital; (2) use a comprehensive approach of community engagement which accounts for culture and historical inequities; and (3) make sustainability a priority.

6. Role of Policy, Systems, and Environmental Change Approaches to Building Healthier Communities

6.1. What Are Policy, Systems, and Environmental Change (PSE) Strategies?

Over the past decade, public health efforts to accelerate chronic disease prevention and reduce health inequities are increasingly focused on policy, systems, and environmental (PSE) approaches. PSE strategies employ modifications to written policies, established community/organizational systems, and built environments to improve access and opportunity for healthier behaviors [56]. PSE strategies also appreciate that interventions which target exo-system factors that influence individual health behaviors are more likely to lead to changes that are long-term and sustainable. Collectively, these approaches attend to the socio-ecological influences of health and human behavior that requires practitioners, researchers, policymakers and other stakeholders to understand psychological and social interactions at multiple levels of analysis and transactions between various networks and their relationships to outcomes. Community engagement is an important process and outcome involved in PSE approaches. It facilitates identification of community leaders' knowledge and skills that should inform program and intervention components appropriate to the community context and designed to meet their health needs [57].

Policies, which refer to rules or procedures used to guide the execution of decisions and actions among individuals, exist at within organizations, agencies, and other governing bodies with the intention of producing positive outcomes [58]. Community institutions such as school districts, churches, non-profit organizations, health care organizations, commercial businesses and daycare centers develop and implement policies. Government bodies at the local, state, federal and international levels create policies that guide the activities of individuals and organizations within the jurisdictions they are responsible for governing. Additionally, policies are important for providing guidance to new partnerships and collaborations between entities such as community coalition boards and academic research teams that have come together to address a problem they can solve together more effectively than separate from each other.

Systems change involves changes made to the rules that various institutions, organizations, and agencies for example, that impact their operations and activities. These changes are made within existing infrastructures which may present challenges to successful implementation. For example, large systems that include thousands of individuals, have many smaller agencies or governing units within the larger system and are widely distributed geographically across a state, a country or around the globe, require changes to be carefully planned and executed to insure favorable outcomes [58]. Systems changes and policy changes are often complimentary and can support or hinder the health goals and objectives of the other depending multiple factors. Health care centers, schools, neighborhood clinics, and community service boards are examples of systems that can and often undergo changes that are designed to strengthen the health outcomes of individuals, families and communities they are responsible to serve.

Environmental change is imperative to strengthening communities. There are many types of physical environments that persons engage on a daily basis that can have a significant impact on their health outcomes including homes, community centers, prisons and grocery stores, for example. While a person may determine that they need to change their behavior to achieve a desired health outcome, examination of environments they frequent may reveal barriers or facilitators of that particular change that are not always readily apparent or observable. From sidewalks in communities designed to increase physical interactions between residents, to prisons that are designed to reduce the need for physical interactions to maintain control of incarcerated individuals, environmental changes can have lasting positive or negative effects on the health of persons within these spaces [58].

6.2. A Paradigm Shift

In The Institute of Medicine's (IOM) landmark report—*The Future of Public Health*, one conclusion indicated was that the public health system and many of its policies involving assessment, service provision, program implementation and other functions was in disarray [44]. *The Future of the Public's Health*, also published by the IOM in 2002 [59], expands this analysis and emphasizes the need for a population health approach, promotes interdisciplinary partnership and collaboration, and calls for a stronger public health infrastructure within government. There was explicit recognition that the policy, systems and environmental changes are critical in shaping the behaviors of individuals and health risks as well [59].

Throughout the late 1990s and 2000s, leading organizations such as the Centers for Disease Control and Prevention (CDC), Institutes of Medicine (IOM), the Robert Wood Johnson Foundation (RWJF), and the National Institutes of Health (NIH) have called for increased efforts at the state and local levels to advance such approaches. This is evidenced by key investments in community and population-level PSE initiatives made by several major entities including federal government agencies and private philanthropic organizations. Racial and Ethnic Approaches to Community Health (REACH) (1996–present), a national initiative administered by the Centers for Disease Control and Prevention to reduce racial and ethnic health disparities largely by promoting engagement between systems to impact health outcomes among disadvantaged populations. REACH program participants employ CBPR approaches to identify, develop and disseminate evidence based strategies to reduce and ultimately eliminate health disparities experienced by vulnerable communities of color. Strategies include a focus on proper nutrition, physical activity, and tobacco use and exposure include cardiovascular disease, diabetes, obesity and infant mortality. REACH awardees focus more directly on systems and environmental changes than policy change, but many achieve remarkable outcomes including lower smoking prevalence, increased intake of fruits and vegetables, and improving immunization rates [60]. Partnerships between governmental agencies such as school boards and health departments and non-governmental agencies such as churches, non-profit organizations, and businesses represent multi-sector collaborations that create program participants with knowledge, skills and the environmental conditions to make healthier lifestyle choices feasible.

The National Institutes of Health (NIH) has also supported key initiatives that utilize policy, systems, and environmental approaches to positively impact population health. The NIH's Office of Behavioral and Social Science Research (OBSSR) brought together experts from a variety of disciplines including medicine, public health, nursing and social work to create a trans-disciplinary model of evidence based practice [61]. This body refined an evidence based model with an ecological framework that promotes change through engagement of interpersonal, organizational, community and public policy levels within practice and research settings. This effort is a great example of how system thinkers within a variety of disciplines collaborated to create a population-based approach to behavior change that was disseminated within and across disciplines, many of which have historically viewed individual-level change as normal and appropriate. Training modules have been developed for educators and evidence suggests that health care providers who have completed the modules demonstrate improvements in knowledge, attitudes and skills related to evidence-based practice [61].

6.3. Policy, Systems, and Environment Change Exemplars

While PSE strategies are diverse in their design and anticipated outcomes, several important exemplars have been recognized in the literature. Communities have achieved improved access to healthy food options through the development of healthy corner and grocery stores, community gardens, mobile food stores and pantries, and providing incentives for SNAP recipients to purchase fresh produce at locally based farmers markets [62–64]. PSEs that have been employed to increase opportunities for physical activity include Safe Routes to School initiatives, urban design and land use policies such as Complete Streets that promote active transportation, joint use agreements, and policies supporting the integration of brief bouts of physical activity into the standard routine of key community and organizational settings [65]. Reductions in the sale of tobacco products, tobacco use, and reduced exposure to tobacco byproducts (e.g., second hand smoke) have been achieved through the adoption of tobacco retail permitting, smoke-free business, school, and multi-unit housing policies [65,66]. Significant efforts have been made to systematically link high-risk community residents to preventive services and community-based wellness assets through: (1) employment of community health workers (CHWs) and other lay health promoters; and (2) leveraging of health information technology to identify high-risk patients and facilitate warm referrals [67–69].

6.4. Opportunities for Community Engaged Leadership in Policy, Systems, and Environment Changes

PSE strategies are nuanced and may require considerable investment in time and resources to achieve maximum impact. Effective, sustainable PSE strategies require collective action among diverse stakeholders, community buy-in, and constant communication to ensure all parties involved are operating from a unified action agenda. Thus, there are ample opportunities for community members and advocates to demonstrate leadership toward the successful adoption, implementation, and evaluation of PSE strategies. Lyn and colleagues [70] identify several key activities associated with PSE: (1) assess the social and political environment; (2) engage, educate, and collaborate with key stakeholders; (3) identify and frame the problem; (4) utilize available evidence; (5) identify policy solutions; and (6) build support and political will. Additional opportunities may arise through the PSE implementation process, and when evaluating PSE feasibility, impact on behaviors and attitudes, and effectiveness in mitigating deleterious health outcomes. We illustrate these crucial opportunities for community leadership by describing two emerging PSEs strategies being facilitated by the Morehouse School of Medicine REACH HI Initiative; Healthy Corner Stores and Complete Streets.

The REACH HI PSE initiative addresses existing PSEs that have contributed to the development of community environments that are barriers to healthy eating and physical activity. In the early 1960s federal transportation policies led to the construction and completion of the I-75/85 interstate highway connector, which cut through the heart of the City of Atlanta. The interstate divided downtown communities, destroying street grids and the connectivity of these neighborhoods. The impact of this imposing infrastructure and the community dissection it created has been disinvestment by businesses, including food establishments, and the loss of street connectivity that previously supported easier access to healthy foods, transit access, and physical activity. For example, from 1962 to 2006, Neighborhood Planning Unit (NPU)-V experienced an 86% decline in businesses; the number of businesses declined from 178 to 41. In 1962, NPU-V was home to 28 grocery/bakery/meat establishments and fifteen restaurants. By 2006, there were only four restaurants and five grocery/bakery/meat stores. As a result of the large loss of businesses and food establishments, corner stores emerged to serve as primary food sources for many in the community. These stores often offer food products that are energy dense but lacking in nutritional quality (e.g., high fat, high sugar). Efforts implemented in this initiative seek to counteract these challenges through conversion of corners stores to provide access to healthy foods and through policies that promote Complete Streets that are safe, connected, and supportive of physical activity.

Community-based participatory approaches were employed to conduct initial community health needs assessments and asset mapping project across several Atlanta NPUs in 2010–2011 and 2013. The assessments were led by a multi-sector coalition of Morehouse School of Medicine investigators, local community health organizations (e.g., United Way of Greater Atlanta), and a governance body comprised of local community residents and elected NPU chairs (Community Coalition Board). The most frequently cited health concerns identified through primary data included high blood pressure, diabetes and overweight/obesity. Among the common causes identified for these concerns were "stores without fresh fruits and vegetables", "access and knowledge of healthy foods", and "lack of affordable and healthy food and exercise options". These concerns laid the foundation for the development of the Healthy Corner Stores and Complete Streets initiatives currently in effect. The Healthy Corner Store initiative seeks to recruit up to 21 local corner stores to enhance their provisions of fruits, vegetables, whole grain options, and low fat food options. The Complete Streets initiative intends to galvanize community support towards the advancement of Complete Streets policy adoption in five NPUs by 2017. All activities within both initiatives must be presented and endorsed by the local CCB prior to execution. Two community-based organizations are responsible for steering community engagement efforts and facilitating communications between community residents and academic investigators. Seasoned community health workers have been strategically employed to identify and map prospective corner stores; assess neighborhood infrastructure hazards (e.g., broken sidewalks, hazardous road conditions, *etc.*); identify existing Complete Streets and other infrastructure projects underway; and assist academic investigators with tailoring Corner Store community awareness and educational materials to best resonate with community stakeholders.

Although community leadership opportunities in employing PSE strategies are plentiful, some important key considerations must be acknowledged. PSEs must be in alignment with community stakeholders' established needs, and community must be amenable to the proposed systems changes and environmental modifications being proposed. Cooperation across diverse sectors (with sometimes divergent agendas) is necessary to fully realize certain PSE strategies.

7. Toward Advancing Health Equity

Public health entities play a major role in reducing health inequities particularly by increasing resources for disadvantaged communities through various programs and by providing a trained workforce to educate these persons. For example, use of community health worker (CHW) and/or patient navigator models has increased in popularity around the globe since the 1980s, which has improved access to health care for underserved communities, supported efficiency in helping people with chronic illnesses to prioritize health management, engaged primary care services, and used preventive care services [71]. Section 5313 of the Patient Protection and Affordable Care Act (PPACA), Subtitle B—Innovations in the Health Care Work Force—recognizes CHWs as essential members of the health care delivery team; and Subtitle D—Enhancing Health Care Workforce Education and Training—indicated that the Centers for Disease Control and Prevention may be significant in facilitating community based efforts to promote health-seeking behaviors in underserved areas.

Health equity is "attainment of the highest level of health for all people" [9]. Lessons that continue to be learned from clinical practice, research, prevention initiatives, and advocacy to inform health policies each has unique yet complementary implications for approaches to improve health equity. There is value in examining successful models that have been implemented in various international regions that may inform models in the U.S. There is a need to more closely examine the significance and benefits of utilizing models of comprehensive, multi-disciplinary, culturally-tailored, patient-centered, and integrative health care delivery systems. For example, integration of behavioral health into primary care may yield positive outcomes and benefits at patient, provider, and clinic/system levels [72]. Also, this approach may help to improve access to quality health care in other countries, especially those with large rural populations that experience significant disparities in health and mental health. Furthermore, it may lead to gains in the development of conceptual frameworks to help reduce stigma in mental health help-seeking and treatment, as well as strategies for reducing disparities in health. Concerning research, innovative community-based, bio-medical, clinical and translational investigations are needed. These research studies must explore the complexities and intersection of multi-dimensional factors, bio-psycho-social issues, and cultural topics that help to elucidate emic and etic considerations about diverse groups. Better dissemination of research outcomes/findings to and from various local, national, and international communities by using inventive strategies will help to promulgate information to promote health. Furthermore, it is critical that prevention, intervention efforts, and health educational programs use bi-directional science discovery, evidence-based models, and intentional community engagement to encourage behaviors and practices that advance improvements in health. Working collaboratively with scholars, researchers and public health care professionals from international communities *versus* simply gathering data from their communities is a critical step in nurturing trust, strengthening credibility, and building global partnerships. Another vital ideal to consider for improving health equity is advocacy and strategic efforts to inform health policies. We have a responsibility to respond when: (1) an issue/topic (*i.e.*, health literacy) is identified but there is no policy to address it; (2) a policy is in place but it needs modification because it is ineffective or has yielded undesired outcomes; (3) a policy is in place but there are barriers to implementation (*i.e.*, health information technology in underserved communities); and (4) gaps that exists between science, policies, and cultural norms that deem the conducting impact analyses (*i.e.*, breastfeeding in the workplace).

Community engaged policy, systems and environmental approaches to improving the health of communities belong to an evolving public health approach that recognizes the importance of focusing on population health. As PSE approaches began to emerge in the late 1990s, particularly within public health, increased recognition and acknowledgement of forces that impact individual health behaviors and outcomes was embraced by stakeholders in medicine, public health, behavioral health and other sectors. This shift in thinking about how to create the conditions that support healthier communities through PSE approaches was supported by local, regional and national government agencies, faith-based, education, NGOs, and other organizations. Partnerships were formed and implementation science was developed to create an evidence base that revealed positive outcomes at the individual, family, and community level in a variety of areas including cardiovascular disease, obesity, diabetes, and hypertension.

We acknowledge that there are challenges to successful implementation of PSE approaches to pressing public health problems such as limited resources and funding. Limitations in available resources may present barriers at various levels for private and public sectors. Moreover, community needs may be identified, yet significant funding to support changes that could be sustainable are difficult to achieve. However, communities press forward, identifying creative and innovative solutions that maximize the skills, knowledge and experience emerging from partnerships that are community-based, egalitarian and promote consensus building. The ultimate goal of community-engaged approaches framed by PSE approaches under ethical leadership is improved community health. Increased utilization of focused, multi-dimensional, inter-sectoral strategies creates the opportunity for a larger positive impact on vulnerable and disadvantaged communities. Leadership that combines evidence based research and programming activities with a collaborative partnership with community members forms the basis of effective mechanisms to build healthier communities. Moreover, developing culturally centered tools and providing communities with educational resources to bolster knowledge and a sense of ownership of their communities, facilitates sustainability such that communities are empowered and mobilized.

Ethical leadership for community health promotion is an integral and central component of addressing health inequities; and stimulating positive change among policy makers and decision-makers. Perhaps, providing a cost-effectiveness and/or cost savings argument that can simultaneously strengthen communities on a systemic level that builds a sustainable infrastructure is one strategic method. This may be particularly relevant concerning the equitable distribution of resources to support health education, creating a workforce of persons that target underserved communities, increasing awareness about the role of social determinants of health among bourgeoning professionals, and working collaboratively with communities. It is imperative that we actively embrace the opportunities before us to respond to Dr. Martin Luther King's proclamation to the Medical Committee for Human Rights in 1966 that "of all the forms of inequality, injustice in health care is the most shocking and inhumane" which starts with building healthier communities.

8. Conclusions

Researchers, public health professionals, clinicians, community members, and policy makers have distinct responsibilities to ensure the health and well-being of individuals, families, and communities. Collectively, through integrity-ethical based leadership, we can promote the reduction health disparities and advance health equity.

Acknowledgments: (1) David Satcher-16th U.S. Surgeon General; Founding Director and Senior Advisor of the Satcher Health Leadership Institute at Morehouse School of Medicine; (2) The project described is supported by the National Institute on Minority Health and Health Disparities (NIMHD) Grant Number U54MD008173, a component of the National Institutes of Health (NIH) and Its contents are solely the responsibility of the authors and do not necessarily represent the official views of NIMHD or NIH; and (3) grant from the Centers for Disease Control and Prevention, Racial and Ethnic Approaches to Community Health (REACH).

Author Contributions: All authors contributed equally towards the development and writing of this article. Each author brings a myriad of experience in community-based engagement and community-based participatory research approaches.

Conflicts of Interest: The authors declare no conflict of interest.

Abbreviations

CBPA	Community-Based Participatory Approach
CBPR	Community-Based Participatory Research
CCB	Community Coalition Board
CDC	Centers for Disease Control and Prevention
IOM	Institute of Medicine
NIH	National Institutes of Health
NPU	Neighborhood Planning Unit
PRC	Prevention Research Center
PSE	Policy, System, and Environmental
RWJF	Robert Wood Johnson Foundation

References

1. Steven H. Woolf, and Laudan Aron, eds. *U.S. Health in International Perspective: Shorter Lives, Poorer Health*. Washington: National Academies Press, 2013.
2. World Health Organization. "Health Manpower Requirements for the Achievement of Health for All by the Year 2000 through Primary Health Care." Paper presented at WHO Expert Committee, Geneva, Switzerland, 12–16 December 1983. Available online: http://apps.who.int/iris/bitstream/10665/ 39110/1/WHO_TRS_717.pdf (accessed on 15 November 2015).
3. U.S. Department of Health and Human Services. *Mental Health: Culture, Race, and Ethnicity—A Supplement to Mental Health: A Report of the Surgeon General*; Rockville: U.S. Department of Health and Human Services, Substance Abuse and Mental Health Services Administration, Center for Mental Health Services, 2001.
4. Michael Marmot, Sharon Friel, Ruth Bell, Tanja A.J. Houweling, and Sebastian Taylor. "Closing the gap in a generation: Health equity through action on the social determinants of health." *The Lancet* 372 (2008): 1661–69.
5. Centers for Disease Control and Prevention. "Health Disparities and Inequalities Report." *Morbidity and Mortality Weekly Report* 62 (2013): 1–187.
6. Annelle B. Primm, Melba J.T. Vasquez, Robert A. Mays, Doreleena Sammons-Posey, Lela R. McKnight-Eily, Letitia R. Presley-Cantrell, Lisa C. McGuire, Daniel P. Chapman, and Geraldine S. Perry. "The role of public health in addressing racial and ethnic disparities in mental health and mental illness." *Preventing Chronic Disease* 7 (2010): A20. Available online: http://www.cdc.gov/pcd/issues/2010/jan/09_0125.htm (accessed on 15 November 2015).
7. Andrew L. Dannenberg, Howard Frumkin, and Richard J. Jackson. *Making Healthy Places: Designing and Building for Health, Well-Being, and Sustainability*, 1st ed. Washington: Island Press, 2011.
8. Mary M. Lee. "Promising Strategies for Building Healthy Communities for All." *National Civic Review* 103 (2014): 13–17.

9. U.S. Department of Health & Human Services. "HHS Action Plan to Reduce Racial and Ethnic Health Disparities: A Nation Free of Disparities in Health and Health Care." 2011. Available online: http:// minorityhealth.hhs.gov/npa/files/plans/hhs/hhs_plan_complete.pdf (accessed on 15 November 2015).
10. Jennifer H. Lee, Ritu Sadana, and the Commission on Social Determinants of Health Knowledge Networks, eds. *Improving Equity in Health by Addressing Social Determinants*. Geneva: World Health Organization, 2011.
11. Centers for Disease Control and Prevention. *National Diabetes Statistics Report: Estimates of Diabetes and Its Burden in the United States, 2014*. Atlanta: US Department of Health and Human Services, 2014.
12. Centers for Disease Control and Prevention. *National Diabetes Fact Sheet: National Estimates and General Information on Diabetes and Prediabetes in the United States, 2011*. Atlanta: U.S. Department of Health and Human Services, Centers for Disease Control and Prevention, 2011.
13. American Diabetes Association. "Economic costs of diabetes in the U.S. in 2002." *Diabetes Care* 26 (2003): 917–32.
14. American Diabetes Association. "Economic costs of diabetes in the U.S. in 2007." *Diabetes Care* 31 (2008): 596–615.
15. Meredith Minkler, and Nina Wallerstein, eds. *Community-Based Participatory Research for Health: From Process to Outcomes*. Hoboken: John Wiley & Sons, 2011.
16. Judith K. Ockene, Elizabeth A. Edgerton, Steven M. Teutsch, Lucy N. Marion, Therese Miller, Janice L. Genevro, Carol J. Loveland-Cherry, Jonathan E. Fielding, and Peter A. Briss. "Integrating evidence-based clinical and community strategies to improve health." *American Journal of Preventive Medicine* 32 (2007): 244–52.
17. Ilene Morof Lubkin, and Pamala D. Larsen. *Chronic Illness: Impact and Interventions*. Burlington: Jones & Bartlett Learning, 2006.
18. Jerome Sarris, Steven Moylan, David A. Camfield, M.P. Pase, David Mischoulon, Michael Berk, F.N. Jacka, and Isaac Schweitzer. "Complementary medicine, exercise, meditation, diet, and lifestyle modification for anxiety disorders: A review of current evidence." *Evidence-Based Complementary and Alternative Medicine* 2012 (2012): 1–20.
19. Felice N. Jacka, Julie A. Pasco, Arnstein Mykletun, Lana J. Williams, Allison Hodge, Sharleen O'Reilly, Mark A. Kotowicz, Michael Berk, and Geoffrey C. Nicholson. "Association of Western and traditional diets with depression and anxiety in women." *American Journal of Psychiatry* 167 (2010): 305–11.
20. Bruce Bolam, Robert West, and David Gunnell. "Does smoking cessation cause depression and anxiety? Findings from the ATTEMPT cohort." *Nicotine & Tobacco Research* 13 (2011): 209–14.
21. Michael J. Zvolensky, Laura E. Gibson, Anka A. Vujanovic, Kristin Gregor, Amit Bernstein, Christopher Kahler, C.W. Legues, Richard A. Brown, and Matthew T. Feldner. "Impact of posttraumatic stress disorder on early smoking lapse and relapse during a self-guided quit attempt among community-recruited daily smokers." *Nicotine & Tobacco Research* 10 (2008): 1415–27.

22. Justin Jagosh, Ann C. Macaulay, Pierre Pluye, Jon Salsberg, Paula L. Bush, Jim Henderson, Erin Sirett, Geoff Wong, Margaret Cargo, Carol P. Herbert, and *et al*. "Uncovering the benefits of participatory research: Implications of a realist review for health research and practice." *Milbank Quarterly* 90 (2012): 311–46.
23. Margaret Cargo, and Shawna L. Mercer. "The value and challenges of participatory research: Strengthening its practice [Review]." *Annual Review of Public Health* 29 (2008): 325–50.
24. Barbara A. Israel, Amy J. Schulz, Edith A. Parker, and Adam B. Becker. "Review of community-based research: Assessing partnership approaches to improve public health." *Annual Review of Public Health* 19 (1998): 173–202.
25. Barbara A. Israel, Eugenia Eng, Amy J. Schulz, Edith A. Parker, and David Satcher. *Methods in Community-Based Participatory Research for Health*. San Francisco: Jossey-Bass, 2005.
26. Ann C. Macaulay, Treena Delormier, Alex M. McComber, Edward J. Cross, Louise P. Potvin, Gilles Paradis, Rhonda L. Kirby, Chantal Saad-Haddad, and Serge Desrosiers. "Desrosiers. Participatory research with native community of Kahnawake creates innovative code of research ethics." *Canadian journal of public health* 89 (1998): 105–8.
27. Liam R. O'Fallon, and Allen Dearry. "Community-based participatory research as a tool to advance environmental health sciences." *Environmental Health Perspectives* 110 (2002): 155–59.
28. Sarena D. Seifer, and Sarah Sisco. "Mining the challenges of CBPR for improvements in urban health." *Journal of Urban Health* 83 (2006): 981–84.
29. Michele L. Allen, Kathleen Culhane-Pera, Shannon Pergament, and Kathleen T. Call. "Facilitating research faculty participation in CBPR: Development of a model based on key informant interviews." *Clinical and Translational Science* 3 (2010): 233–38.
30. Jennifer A. Sandoval, Julie Lucero, John Oetzel, Magdalena Avila, Lorenda Belone, Marjorie Mau, Cynthia Pearson, Greg Tafoya, Bonnie Duran, Lisbeth Iglesias Rios, and *et al*. "Process and outcome constructs for evaluating community-based participatory research projects: A matrix of existing measures." *Health Education Research* 27 (2012): 680–90.
31. Nina Wallerstein, and Bonnie Duran. "Community-based participatory research contributions to intervention research: The intersection of science and practice to improve health equity." *American Journal of Public Health* 100 (2010): S40–46.
32. Rebecca S. Miller, Larry A. Green, Paul A. Nutting, Lyle Petersen, Linda Stewart, Guillermo Marshall, and Deborah S. Main. "Human immunodeficiency virus seroprevalence in community-based primary care practices, 1990–1992. A report from the Ambulatory Sentinel Practice Network." *Archives of Family Medicine* 4 (1995): 1042–47.
33. Daniel S. Blumenthal. "A community coalition board creates a set of values for community-based research." *Preventing Chronic Disease* 3 (2006): A16.
34. Robert G. Bringle, and Julie A. Hatcher. "Campus-Community Partnerships: The Terms of Engagement." *Journal of Social Issues* 58 (2002): 503–16.
35. George Caspar Homans. *Social Behavior*. New York: Harcourt Brace and World, 1961.

36. John W. Thibaut, and Harold H. Kelley. *The Social Psychology of Groups*. New York: Wiley, 1959.
37. Daniel Blumenthal. "'How do you start working with a community?' Section 4a of 'Challenges in Improving Community Engagement in Research', Chapter 5 of The Clinical and Translational Science Awards Community Engagement Key Function Committee Task Force on the Principles of Community Engagement." In *Principles of Community Engagement*, 2nd ed. Washington: U.S. Department of Health and Human Services, 2011.
38. Akintobi T. Henry, Lisa Goodin, Ella H. Trammel, David Collins, and Daniel Blumenthal. "'How do you set up and maintain a community advisory board?' Section 4b of 'Challenges in Improving Community Engagement in Research', Chapter 5 of The Clinical and Translational Science Awards Community Engagement Key Function Committee Task Force on the Principles of Community Engagement." In *Principles of Community Engagement*, 2nd ed. Washington: U.S. Department of Health and Human Services, 2011.
39. Tabia Henry Akintobi, Nazeera Dawood, and Daniel S. Blumenthal. "An Academic-Public Health Department Partnership for Education, Research, Practice and Governance." *Journal of Public Health Management & Practice* 20 (2014): 310–14.
40. Tabia Henry Akintobi, Lisa Goodin, and LaShawn Hoffman. "Morehouse School of Medicine Prevention Research Center: Collaborating with neighborhoods to develop community-based participatory approaches to address health disparities in Metropolitan Atlanta." *Atlanta Medicine: Journal of the Medical Association of Atlanta* 84 (2013): 14–17.
41. Kirsten C. Rodgers, Tabia Henry Akintobi, Winifred Wilkins Thompson, Donoria Evans, Cam Escoffery, and Michelle C. Kegler. "A model for strengthening collaborative research capacity: Illustrations from the Atlanta Clinical Translational Science Institute." *Health Education and Behavior* 41 (2014): 267–74.
42. John Hatch, Nancy Moss, Ama Saran, and Letitia Presley-Cantrell. "Community research: Partnership in black communities." *American Journal of Preventive Medicine* 9 (1993): 27–31.
43. Ronald L. Braithwaite, Sandra E. Taylor, and John N. Austin. *Building Health Coalitions in the Black Community*. Thousand Oaks: Sage Publications, 1999.
44. Bailus Walker Jr. "The future of public health: The institute of medicine's 1988 report." *Journal of Public Health Policy* 10 (1989): 19–31.
45. Walter E. Fluker. *Ethical Leadership: The Quest for Character, Civility, and Community*. Minneapolis: Augsburg Fortress, 2009.
46. Fitzhugh Mullan, Candice Chen, Stephen Petterson, Gretchen Kolsky, and Michael Spagnola. "The social mission of medical education: Ranking the schools." *Annals of Internal Medicine* 152 (2010): 804–11.
47. J. Scott Carter, and Shannon K. Carter. "Place matters: The impact of place of residency on racial attitudes among regional and urban migrants." *Social Science Research* 47 (2014): 165–77.

48. Katherine Schaff, Alexandra Desautels, Rebecca Flournoy, Keith Carson, Teresa Drenick, Darlene Fujii, Anna Lee, Jessica Luginbuhl, Mona Mena, Amy Shrago, and et al. "Addressing the social determinants of health through the Alameda County, California, place matters policy initiative." *Public Health Reports* 128 (2013): 48–53. Available online: http://www.ncbi.nlm.nih.gov/pubmed/24179279 (accessed on 15 November 2015).
49. Vedette R. Gavin, Eileen L. Seeholzer, Janeen B. Leon, Sandra Byrd Chappelle, and Ashwini R. Sehgal. "If we build it, we will come: A model for community-led change to transform neighborhood conditions to support healthy eating and active living." *American Journal of Public Health* 105 (2015): 1072–77.
50. Sandra A. Austin, and Nancy Claiborne. "Faith wellness collaboration: A community-based approach to address type II diabetes disparities in an African-American community." *Social Work in Health Care* 50 (2011): 360–75.
51. Carolyn Cannuscio, Eva Bugos, Shari Hersh, David A. Asch, and Eve E. Weiss. "Using art to amplify youth voices on housing insecurity." *American Journal of Public Health* 102 (2012): 10–12.
52. Laura Horne, Katie Miller, Sandra Silva, and Lori Anderson. "Implementing the ACHIEVE model to prevent and reduce chronic disease in rural Klickitat County, Washington." *Preventing Chronic Disease* 10 (2013): E56.
53. Samina Raja, Michael Ball, Justin Booth, Philip Haberstro, and Katherine Veith. "Leveraging neighborhood-scale change for policy and program reform in Buffalo, New York." *American Journal of Preventive Medicine* 37 (2009): S352–60.
54. Thomas A. LaVeist, William C. Richardson, Nancy F. Richardson, Rachel Relosa, and Nadia Sawaya. "The COA360: A tool for assessing the cultural competency of health care organizations." *Journal of Healthcare Management* 53 (2008): 257–66.
55. Ronald L. Braithwaite, Sandra E. Taylor, and Henrie M. Treadwell, eds. *Health Issues in the Black Community*. Hoboken: John Wiley & Sons, Inc., 2009.
56. Phyllis Nichols, Ann Ussery-Hall, Shannon Griffin-Blake, and Alyssa Easton. "The evolution of the steps program, 2003–2010: Transforming the federal public health practice of chronic disease prevention." *Preventing Chronic Disease* 9 (2012): 11–22.
57. American Cancer Society. "Policy, Systems, and Environmental Change: Resource Guide, 2015". Available online: http://smhs.gwu.edu/cancercontroltap/sites/cancercontroltap/files/PSE_Resource_Guide_FINAL_05.15.15.pdf (accessed on 15 November 2015).
58. The Health Trust. "What Is Policy, Systems and Environmental (PSE) Change? 2012". Available online: http://healthtrust.org/wp-content/uploads/2013/11/2012-12-28-Policy_Systems_and_Environmental_Change.pdf (accessed on 8 November 2015).
59. Institute of Medicine of the National Academies. *The Future of the Public's Health in the 21st Century*. Washington: The National Academies Press, 2003.

60. Centers for Disease Control and Prevention. "Investments in Community Health: Racial & Ethnic Approaches to Community Health (REACH)." 2014. Available online: http://www.cdc.gov/nccdphp/dch/programs/reach/pdf/2-reach_factsheet-for-web.pdf (accessed on 15 November 2015).
61. Robin P. Newhouse, and Bonnie Spring. "Interdisciplinary evidence-based practice: Moving from silos to synergy." *Nursing Outlook* 58 (2010): 309–17.
62. Hannah G. Lawman, Stephanie Vander Veur, Giridhar Mallya, Tara A. McCoy, Alexis Wojtanowski, Lisa Colby, Timothy A. Sanders, Michelle R. Lent, Brianna A. Sandoval, and Sandy Sherman. "Changes in quantity, spending, and nutritional characteristics of adult, adolescent and child urban corner store purchases after an environmental intervention." *Preventive Medicine* 74 (2015): 81–85.
63. Erica Cavanaugh, Sarah Green, Giridhar Mallya, Ann Tierney, Colleen Brensinger, and Karen Glanz. "Changes in food and beverage environments after an urban corner store intervention." *Preventive Medicine* 65 (2014): 7–12.
64. Daniela Guitart, Catherine Pickering, and Jason Byrne. "Past results and future directions in urban community gardens research." *Urban Forestry & Urban Greening* 11 (2012): 364–73.
65. Rebecca Bunnell, Dara O'Neil, Robin Soler, Rebecca Payne, Wayne H. Giles, Janet Collins, Ursula Bauer, and Communities Putting Prevention to Work Program Group. "Fifty communities putting prevention to work: Accelerating chronic disease prevention through policy, systems and environmental change." *Journal of Community Health* 37 (2012): 1081–90.
66. Nicole Coxe, Whitney Webber, Janie Burkhart, Bonnie Broderick, Ken Yeager, Laura Jones, and Marty Fenstersheib. "Use of tobacco retail permitting to reduce youth access and exposure to tobacco in Santa Clara County, California." *Preventive Medicine* 67 (2014): S46–50.
67. Robina Josiah Willock, Robert M. Mayberry, Fengxia Yan, and Pamela Daniels. "Peer Training of Community Health Workers to Improve Heart Health among African American Women." *Health Promotion Practice* 16 (2015): 63–71.
68. Sarah Klein, Martha Hostetter, and Douglas McCarthy. "A Vision for using digital health technologies to empower consumers and transform the US Health Care System, 2014". Available online: http://www.commonwealthfund.org/~/media/files/publications/fund-report/2014/oct/1776_klein_vision_using_digital_hlt_tech_v2.pdf (accessed on 15 November 2015).
69. Daniel S. Blumenthal. *Community-Based Participatory Health Research: Issues, Methods, and Translation to Practice*. New York: Springer Publishing Company, 2013.
70. Rodney Lyn, Semra Aytur, Tobey A. Davis, Amy A. Eyler, Kelly R. Evenson, Jamie F. Chriqui, Angie L. Cradock, Karin Valentine Goins, Jill Litt, and Ross C. Brownson. "Policy, systems, and environmental approaches for obesity prevention: A framework to inform local and state action." *Journal of Public Health Management and Practice* 19 (2013): S23–33.

71. Moises Perez, Sally E. Findley, Miriam Mejia, and Jacqueline Martinez. "The impact of community health worker training and programs in NYC." *Journal of Health Care for the Poor and Underserved* 17 (2006): 26–43.
72. Amy M. Bauer, Vanessa Azzone, Howard H. Goldman, Laurie Alexander, Jürgen Unützer, Brenda Coleman-Beattie, and Richard G. Frank. "Implementation of Collaborative Depression Management at Community-Based Primary Care Clinics: An Evaluation." *Psychiatric Services* 62 (2011): 1047–53.

Integrated Social Housing and Health Care for Homeless and Marginally-Housed Individuals: A Study of the Housing and Homelessness Steering Committee in Ontario, Canada

Kristy Buccieri

Abstract: Homelessness is a complex social issue that requires a coordinated systems approach. In recent years, Canada has seen an emergence of integrated care, the joining of health care and social care, to address the needs of homeless persons. This article documents the findings of open-ended interviews with eleven members of the central east Ontario Housing and Homelessness Framework Steering Committee, comprised of service managers and the Local Health Integration Network. As the system planners for social housing and health care, respectively, members of the group work together to align system approaches for homeless persons. Research by this group identified three challenges of collaborating—their different histories and legislation, varied accountability structures, and differing roles and responsibilities within the central east region of Ontario. The study findings indicate that developing a joint document to guide the work was a process through which members began to work through these differences.

> Reprinted from *Soc. Sci.* Cite as: Buccieri, K. Integrated Social Housing and Health Care for Homeless and Marginally-Housed Individuals: A Study of the Housing and Homelessness Steering Committee in Ontario, Canada. *Soc. Sci.* **2016**, 5, 15.

1. Introduction

In the fall of 2014, the central-east region of Ontario began a ground-breaking initiative that brought municipal service managers from four regions together with the local health system planner—the Central East Local Health Integration Network (CE-LHIN)—to form a joint ten-year Housing and Homelessness Steering Committee. This undertaking is an innovative community-based approach to integrated care for homeless and marginally-housed individuals. While integrated care, the joining of health care and social care, is well-documented in the United Kingdom [1,2], it remains a relatively new approach in Canada and across North America. This article details the findings of an ethnographic study of the Housing and Homelessness Steering Committee from the central-east region of Ontario, which comprises approximately 882,000 people and is positioned to the immediate northeast of Toronto. Through this Steering Committee, members jointly attempt to design social housing and health-based programs and initiatives in a coordinated manner for homeless and marginally-housed community members.

The Steering Committee provides an opportunity to study an integrated care initiative as it forms and evolves over time. At the time of the research, conducted in the spring and summer of 2015, the Steering Committee had been meeting every two months for approximately one year. In that time, they developed a guiding document that outlined the committee's purpose, strategic aim, member roles, guiding principles, and terms of reference. The creation of this document was an important output of the committee, as it represented the first time the municipal service managers and the CE-LHIN had formally worked together to address issues of housing, homelessness, and health for community members living in the central east region of Ontario. As the system planners, funders, and administrators for housing and homelessness programs in their communities, representatives of four municipal service managers came together in person and on paper with representatives from the CE-LHIN, the system planners and funders for local health initiatives. This jointly-created document marked a critical moment; it provided tangible support for—and a commitment to—providing integrated care for homeless and marginally-housed individuals within these communities (see Figure 1).

The development of this group is important, not only because it provides documented evidence for integrated care, but because it brings together individuals who are working under different provincial ministries, funded through different initiatives, and governed through different policies and pieces of legislation. Until this committee began, representatives from the municipal service managers and the CE-LHIN had never worked directly together. The regions in this study all experience a demand for affordable housing that outweighs the supply. For instance, in the respective regions: less than 1% of new housing stock built between 2000–2009 was rental [3], rental housing is described as limited and not affordable to low-income households [4], tenants comprise 19% of households but only 5% of new housing stock is rental [5], and over 1500 applicants are on the social housing waiting list [6]. The formation of the Steering Committee is an attempt to collectively address the issue of social housing and to align funding efforts with the CE-LHIN.

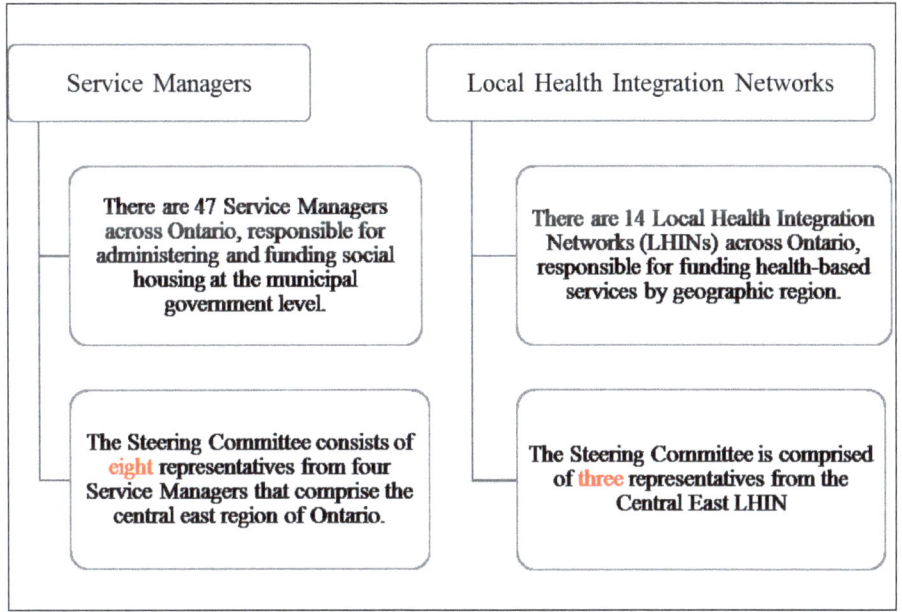

Figure 1. Overview of the Steering Committee members, including representatives from four municipal service managers and the Central East LHIN.

In this article, I begin by providing an overview of the literature on homelessness in Canada, with a particular focus on Ontario, and discuss the methodology of the study. Subsequently, I detail the evolution of municipal service managers and the CE-LHIN and examine the three main challenges that members identified in working together—their differing histories and legislation, varied accountability structures, and different orientations toward responsibilities and roles in the central east region of Ontario. I conclude the article with a discussion of how the members jointly created a document to lead their work, a process they noted allowed them to identify and begin to work through these three challenges. The discussion is intended to inform the efforts of others working collaboratively on integrated care for homelessness and marginally housed individuals.

2. Homelessness, Health, and Integrated Care in Canada

The negative effects of homelessness on physical and mental health are well-documented in Canada, for both adults [7,8] and youth [9]. Entry into homelessness is often associated with a sharp decrease in health status [10], with the occurrence of chronic conditions that are caused and/or reinforced by poverty and the street lifestyle [11]. For instance, in one longitudinal study of homeless individuals in the three Canadian cities of Ottawa, Vancouver, and Toronto, researchers found that over 85% of participants reported having at least one chronic health condition [12]. Among the most frequently reported conditions found in one study of 149 homeless persons in Toronto, were fatigue, coughing up phlegm or blood, shortness of breath, night-sweats, chest pain, unexplained weight loss or gain, lung disease, arthritis, hepatitis A, B, or C, and diabetes, among others [13]. Researchers in Canada have found that homeless individuals are at higher risk of traumatic brain injury than the general public [14,15], report high rates of untreated dental conditions, with low incidents of dental visits [16], and often face challenges obtaining stable and nutritious food sources [17,18]. Many homeless individuals report experiencing mental health issues [19], whether clinically diagnosed [12] or a more general sense of loneliness on the street [20]. Substance use is common among homeless individuals in Canada, and in many instances is related to, or complicated by, mental health factors [21,22].

Despite the evidence that shows homeless individuals experience poor physical and mental health outcomes related to living on the street or in unstable conditions, many homeless individuals rate their health as being excellent or very good [13]. In one study from Toronto, Vancouver, and Ottawa, researchers found many homeless and vulnerably-housed participants rated their health as fair or average; here the authors noted that it is important to contextualize these findings with the understanding that participants frame their own health in relation to those of their friends and family who are in similar circumstances [23]. Homeless individuals often do not access preventative medical care services, describing instances of previous health care visits as being dehumanizing and stigmatizing [24]. Forging a chain of trust, particularly within nurse-patient interactions for marginalized populations, is important in creating a welcoming health care setting [25]. Without this trust, feelings of embarrassment and shame have been found to prevent homeless individuals from seeking out medical information, particularly around sexual health issues for young female and transgender youth [26]. The pressing physical and mental health needs of homeless individuals, combined with their low help-seeking behavior, lends support to the placement of accessible services, like public health clinics, in community-based shelters and drop-in centres [27]. However, while many homeless individuals report accessing some form of services [28], research has also found that the institutional cycling of clients through different agencies can contribute to the spread of disease among service users [29,30].

Improving the health and wellness of homeless persons requires a coordinated approach, such that individuals are able to access a range of services and supports without having to cycle through the system in the process. Integrated care involves bringing together health and social supports in a way that supports the client and his/her particular needs at the centre. While integrated care has been defined in different ways, Kodner and Spreeuwenberg offer one definition that is frequently cited. Accordingly, they write:

> Integration is a coherent set of methods and models on the funding, administrative, organisational, service delivery and clinical levels designed to create connectivity, alignment and collaboration within and between the cure and care sectors. The goal of these methods and models is to enhance quality of care and quality of life, consumer satisfaction and system efficiency for patients with complex, long-term problems cutting across multiple services, providers and settings. The result of such multi-pronged efforts to promote integration for the benefit of these special patient groups is called "integrated care" [31].

For homeless individuals, integrated care may involve the coordination of housing, health care provision, and mental health and/or substance use supports.

One example of the integrated care philosophy for homeless individuals in North America, is the proliferation of the Housing First model, which emerged through the work of Dr. Sam Tsemberis and Pathways to Housing in the United States [32]. Housing First is defined within a Canadian context as being:

> ...a recovery-oriented approach to homelessness that involves moving people who experience homelessness into independent and permanent housing as quickly as possible, with no preconditions, and then providing them with additional services and supports as needed. The underlying principle of Housing First is that people are more successful in moving forward with their lives if they are first housed [33].

Housing First is an integrated care approach that connects individuals with supportive housing and case workers who provide transitional assistance and a sense of stability, often with a focus on improving their mental health and wellness.

The Housing First model was implemented in the five Canadian cities of Vancouver, Winnipeg, Toronto, Montréal, and Moncton through the "At Home/Chez Soi" study that operated from 2009–2013 [34]. Through this study, a combined total of 2148 individuals were enrolled in different intervention types, with 1158 placed in the Housing First model. The results of the study strongly indicate that homeless and marginally housed individuals benefit from the combination of housing and integrated supports, like health care provision and mental health/substance use supports. It should be noted, however, that while supported as an integrated approach, the implementation of the Housing First model requires that structural issues be addressed, such as the existing shortage of affordable housing in Ontario [35,36].

A body of Canadian research on supportive housing models that combine subsidized or social housing with accessible supports, shows that the integrated approach to service provision is largely effective. Individual studies have shown that housing combined with supports has a positive effect on health [37], improves outcomes for individuals with serious mental illness [38], improves perceived quality of life [39], increases life satisfaction [40], lowers hospital emergency room visits for adults with mental disorders [41], and reduces the number of days individuals report experiencing alcohol problems [42]. Integrated care models, like Housing First, have been found to be of greatest efficacy when they target the most intensive users of services [38], and when they are supported by staff expertise, multi-service partnerships, and strong leadership [43]. However, research on the accuracy of Housing First success predictive models have found them to be largely ineffective at determining who will maintain stable housing [44].

The health of homeless persons is affected by many factors, with housing status and access to supports being among the most important. Addressing the high rates of chronic health conditions, mental health issues, and substance use found amongst homeless populations in Canada requires a broad social lens that accounts for the multiple factors impacting their health and wellness. While research has shown that not all clinicians working with homeless populations report feeling initially prepared to address the impacts of the social determinants of health on their patients [45], Doran, Misa, and Shah write that:

> Social determinants of health should be central to mainstream discussions and funding decisions about health care. For many patients, a prescription for housing or food is the most powerful one that a physician could write, with health effects far exceeding those of most medications [46].

Integrated models that take a broader social perspective of health care delivery are becoming more common, as they improve patient outcomes and reduce overall costs of service provision [47]. However, even though health care leaders may support these kinds of innovative approaches, the time, funds, and energy required for a relatively small population may not be where they choose to devote their often limited resources [48].

Kodner and Spreeuwenberg note that the effective design and implementation of integrated care may face barriers and bottlenecks in the five interlocking domains of funding, administration, organization, service delivery, and clinical practice [31]. Others, in a collection of essays, have similarly argued that creating integrated care is challenging and must first address issues pertaining to shared budgets between health and care sectors [49,50], the need for strong and informed leadership [51], the creation of (potentially legally binding) documents that guide and frame collaborations [52], and transparency through shared data [53]. Creating strategies that integrate health and social care, while challenging, are particularly important for addressing the complex needs of homeless individuals.

3. Methodology

The study design was influenced by institutional ethnography, as developed and informed through the work of Dorothy Smith [54]. The study involved document review such as municipal housing and homelessness plans [3–6], participant observation, and Steering Committee interviews. Institutional ethnography is a sociological approach that takes texts and documents as an entry point into understanding a given problem. The problematic examined in this study was how the service managers and Central East LHIN organized their relations and interactions with one another, around social housing and health system planning. The guiding question was, "What are the key considerations and challenges that arise in developing a ten-year Housing and Homelessness Framework to guide partnerships and collaboration, according to the Central East LHIN staff and service managers?" The Housing and Homelessness Framework Steering Committee meets in person every two months, in rotating locations throughout the central east region of Ontario. As the Principal Investigator, I attended all seven of the meetings that occurred during the research period, as a participant-observer, and took hand-written research notes. Each meeting lasted approximately 2.5 h.

In the summer of 2015, I conducted semi-structured interviews with all members of the Steering Committee, including three representatives from the CE-LHIN, and two representatives from each of the four municipal service managers. The interviews ranged from one to three hours in length. In three of the regions, service manager interviews were conducted in pairs and in one region interviews were conducted with two members separately. The CE-LHIN interview was conducted with three members, although one member was newer to the Steering Committee and observed more than participated in the interview, creating a paired-interview dynamic much like several of the service managers. In each interview, a guide was used to direct questions but the order of questions was sometimes altered to allow for a more conversational flow. Despite sometimes being in different orders, all participants (whether from a service manager or CE-LHIN) were asked the same questions in five general themes pertaining to their employment role and history; policy and funding context in which they worked; creation of the mandated municipal ten-year housing and homelessness plans; involvement in the Housing and Homelessness Framework Steering Committee; and assistance in creating a timeline of key events and documents shaping their work.

This study was reviewed and approved by Trent University's research ethics board. Participants were provided with the questions in advance and each gave written informed consent. The interviews were audio-recorded and transcribed by the principal investigator and a research assistant. All participants were provided with a copy of the written transcript following the interview and were given thirty days to correct or redact any information they wished. While some minor revisions were made, none of the transcripts were significantly altered from their original texts. All interview transcripts were coded by the Principal Investigator according to the five interview question themes noted above. A table was created in which each response was posted and represented alongside those of other members for each question. I utilized a coding method that involved examining the comparative quotes for similarities, differences, and novel information, as described by Kirby, Greaves, and Reid [55]. To help protect participant anonymity, quotes are attributed only to a CE-LHIN or service manager participant throughout the article, without identifying details provided.

This study does have limitations that should be noted at the outset. First, the Steering Committee is comprised of a small number of representatives (*i.e.*, eleven). While every participant was included in the study and the findings can be considered representative of this particular committee, it is unknown how their composition may differ from other groups of this nature. Second, the committee is comprised of system planners and does not include those with identified lived experience of homelessness and/or front-line service providers. As a planning table, these voices are not represented in the committee or in this study. Finally, the group is in its infancy and the study can only provide an examination of how it has formed over its first year. A longitudinal study that evaluated its progress and impact at the community-level would be a valuable long-term undertaking.

4. Health and Social Housing Sector Collaboration: Identifying Key Challenges

The Homelessness and Housing Framework Steering Committee is comprised of system planners from the Central East Local Health Integration Network and service managers responsible for funding and administering social housing and homelessness programs in their four respective communities. The Steering Committee meets every two months to try and jointly align funding and programming initiatives that affect the health and wellness of homeless and marginally housed individuals. However, despite taking a collective approach to these issues, the members of the Steering Committee are differently positioned based on a number of key factors. Across sectors—whether health or social housing—committee members are governed by their own legislation and are expected to undertake different roles. Further, between and within sectors, accountability and area of responsibility varies. These three factors—legislation, accountability, and roles—are discussed first as factors that align the group members differently, and at times give rise to conflict and/or challenges. In the section that follows, I discuss the measures the committee members have taken to help address and overcome these factors in building a collaborative framework together.

4.1. Legislative and Historical Differences

The province of Ontario provides a novel landscape in which to examine integrated care initiatives like the Housing and Homelessness Framework Steering Committee because the LHINs and service managers are both uniquely Ontario-made through their respective legislation and histories. In the interviews, all participants were asked to speak about the legislative contexts in which they work and to outline the historical evolution of their organizations and roles. While the service managers are all governed by the same pieces of legislation, these do not overlap with the LHIN. The misalignment between the guiding legislation was felt by many participants to be an impediment to integrated work between the health and social housing sectors.

Across Ontario, there are fourteen LHINs, each responsible for health system planning and funding in a designated geographic area, as legislated through the Local Health System Integration Act (LHSIA), 2006 [56]. The introduction of the LHINs in Ontario was met with some public skepticism about their longevity and concern around the term "integration" and what it meant for health care providers. One participant stated that, "I think in the beginning people just didn't know what to make of us and couldn't figure out what we were doing" (CE-LHIN 1). Another participant stated:

> CE-LHIN 2: I think when we started it, people were like, "Oh, here comes the next—or first—wave really of integration." I have been through a few system integrations but it was always the planning entities in the province, and the LHIN was the necessary move to bring planning and funding accountability into one local body…But we did not know if it would stick through governments…It's been three elections, at least, of provincial government that…it's stuck through.

Initial public concerns focused on the word "integration" and what it meant for health service providers:

> CE-LHIN 2: With the word "integration" in our name and that being a new term, there was a lot of discussion about, "What does that mean? Is that a merger? Amalgamation? Cease our service? What is that?" We spent a lot of our time in [the] early days explaining that, absolutely, that is part of the continuum of integration but partnerships, collaborations, transfers, mergers, amalgamations, stop service are all in the [LHSIA] as a continuum.

While some uncertainty remains, the CE-LHIN participants believed that their work is better understood and appreciated today than it had been previously:

> CE-LHIN 1: I think [the public] understand[s] what it means better. There's still some providers that are very frightened by that. I think

the fright comes from believing that they're going to lose their service and their jobs. The opportunity that people see now, that perhaps we saw in the beginning, is the opportunity for the people that they serve. So whereas the planning used to be based on the service, it's now based on the person being served and I think now that people see that, it's kind of renewed the interests of some people who were working in the field.

In comparison to the LHINs, service managers have been operational considerably longer and have also changed and evolved over time. The role began with the federal devolution of social housing to provinces in the 1990s and the subsequent download in Ontario to municipal service managers and District Social Services Administration Boards (DSABs) [57]. Initially created under the Social Housing Reform Act (SHRA), 2000 [58], the service manager role was recently amended and is now legislated through the Housing Services Act (HSA), 2011 [59]. The impacts of federal and provincial downloads are still very much felt today by those in service manager roles. According to one service manager representative interviewed for this project, "...back in 2001 when they transferred housing to the service manager—just a box. Here's a box and a handshake, and I'm serious about that" (SM 1). The history of federal devolutions and provincial downloads have greatly shaped the work of social housing administration in Ontario today. This theme emerged in multiple interviews:

> SM 2: [The legislation and funding procedures identified within them are] overly complicated, I think at this point. And I think the root of the problem is that the devolution was done too quickly and there wasn't enough consolidation at that point and there wasn't enough faith in municipalities that they could do a good job and that may have been appropriate back in the day. Municipalities were terribly resistant to this [download].

> SM 3: It's a very different world since download. There are a lot more procedures, a lot more things written down...certainly there were no service managers, that kind of collaboration between service managers to get things in place. It's a lot more formal and written down, so that hopefully years and years from now, people won't have to go, "Why did that happen?"

> SM 4: One of the interesting things about service managers, and our evolution, is when housing portfolio was downloaded there were a ton of people with lots of—20–30 years'—experience in housing delivery, provincial housing delivery program, that ended up in service manager positions across the province...So we rely on that expertise that is

now imbedded within the service manager role to help create some information, fill the information gaps that sometimes all these young folk don't have.

The two primary pieces of legislation that guide the work of the LHINs and service managers are separate and distinct. However, while this separation may be expected given these two groups operate within different sectors, the LHSIA (*i.e.*, the legislation that created LHINs) was created after the service manager boundaries had long been established and operational. This lack of coordination—and the missed opportunity for alignment—was a source of considerable frustration that was expressed in multiple interviews.

> CE-LHIN 1: With the municipal lens, to a certain extent, we're wandering into territory that we don't really understand, as well as there's some of those old wounds from other processes that we weren't involved in that rear their heads in this process.

> SM 3: The province created the Consolidated Municipal service managers and the DSABs…So why, when they created the LHINs, didn't they try and align that with the service managers? That was created by the province—the same province—so why didn't they align it? Perhaps if they had aligned it, things would have evolved differently.

> SM 2: The geographic boundaries at the province have never been properly addressed. It's a huge project, but the geographic boundaries are used by all ministries and they set up the province in different ways, and there ought to be an approach whereby we always know that we're connected with these five other municipalities, whereas we're not.

The different legislative contexts and historical evolutions of service managers and the LHIN poses a practical challenge to collaborative working relations. For example, the CE-LHIN is also the health system planner for Scarborough, a region of Toronto that is considerably different in geography and population than the other four communities, and as such is not represented on the Steering Committee. An additional challenge is that one of the service manager regions extends beyond the boundaries of the CE-LHIN, causing them to fall within the bounds of two LHINs. The misalignment of provincial boundaries, such that the work of the LHIN does not clearly overlay the work of the service manager communities, is an issue that the Steering Committee members identified in working together on integrated care planning for homeless persons.

4.2. Accountability Structures

Service managers and LHINs are bound by different accountability structures, with the service managers guided by their own municipal elected councils and each LHIN reporting to an appointed board of directors. The nature of the accountability—whether elected or appointed—was described as being an important factor in the reporting relations. According to one CE-LHIN interview participant, the service managers are, "...much closer to the political process than we are. They answer to an elected council, whereas we don't. We have an appointed board, so we don't really have those same pressures" (CE-LHIN 1). The evolution of the service manager role in administering and funding social housing, discussed above, serves to shape the relations with the elected officials to whom they report. This was addressed by one CE-LHIN interview participant who stated:

> CE-LHIN 2: Our municipal partners have had to deal with downloads...They also are still having conversations with their municipal councils discussing the appropriateness of who delivers what, and we have similar conversations but the "who delivers what" and "who's being asked to deliver what" is very at the forefront of their discussions.

While the service managers all report to elected officials, they are each designed and operate independently from one another. One service manager representative stated:

> SM 4: It's a little bit different in every service manager...so it can be different in terms of the reporting. In terms of the broader goals and objectives and the things that we have to do, they're the same because we're falling under the same [legislation]. Just the nuance of council direction and priorities that are set out by those local councils and in terms of the internal arrangement and the reporting, that will be different based on what the infrastructure is within the level of government because we're regional governments.

The nature of the reporting relationship with regional council members is also different across service manager communities. Whereas one service manager representative described the relationship with council members as, "...more of a neighborly relationship. I can sit down and talk to them, we can go out for lunch, there's a comfortable relaxing environment" (SM 1), another service manager from a different region stated, "...when you talk about relationships I think of individual one-on-one relationships, and council is a body of people" (SM 2).

The nature of the accountability and reporting differs between service managers and the LHIN, with elected officials and appointed boards, respectively, in those roles. When working collaboratively together, these differences in accountability structures can produce challenges related to factors such as political sensitivities, operational timelines, and budgetary considerations. The accountability of each party involved in the Steering Committee was a central consideration in moving the group towards a collaborative framework.

4.3. Priorities and Roles

The third identified challenge of collaborating within the Steering Committee was the different nature of the service manager and LHIN roles. Within their individual communities, service managers are responsible for establishing, funding, and administering social housing (among other) programs, while the LHIN serves exclusively in a funding capacity without the administration component. These different functions were noted by several interview participants. According to one service manager representative:

> SM 5: There's an interesting kind of dynamic, in my opinion, in that [service managers] are immersed in our community and we have community partners that we're trying to do this work with, but we have a dual role of we are providing service and we are funding service and the LHIN has only the role of funding service. But, at least in this forum we are able to talk funder to funder.

Beyond the different roles, as administrators and/or funders, the Steering Committee members also bring to the table their unique positions and priorities. In particular, the CE-LHIN interest extends broadly across the central east region of Ontario, while service managers are concerned with their individual municipalities. As a planning table, the differently aligned interests of the parties emerged as a notable challenge that needed to be considered and addressed. The difference in priorities was noted by CE-LHIN and service manager interview participants:

> CE-LHIN 2: [service manager] interests are most directed to their own. They're less interested in knowing what another municipality has. We're very interested to know how the different municipalities are using similar pots of money. That's not so much their concern, other than sometimes if it's problem solving for them.

> SM 4: There's one LHIN and then there's the service managers, which are multiples...And so what we're trying to do is create some more, better balance in the system across the communities but we're still coming at it from a service manager perspective. We're coming at this from our individual service managers and not one-to-one...We're not coming at it as service manager/LHIN. We're coming at it from service managers *and* LHIN, which must make it very difficult for them because they're the ones trying to do the balance...I think that's an important piece of the structure, that it's 4:1.

Entering into a collaborative Steering Committee with different roles and service area priorities was a challenge that service managers and the CE-LHIN had to collectively address and attempt to overcome.

5. Working through Key Challenges: Drafting a Guiding Framework Document

The Steering Committee was formed with the recognition that key challenges existed, stemming from their historical and legislative differences, accountability structures, and varied priorities and roles. Members sought to address these challenges through the joint creation of a guiding document. Throughout the first year, the Steering Committee devoted 20 to 30 min at each meeting to collaboratively drafting a guiding principles and terms of reference document that outlined their work together [60]. The final product is an eight-page document that will be reviewed annually and contains sections on the Steering Committee's purpose and strategic aim, member roles, legislative and policy context, guiding principles, terms of reference, and approvals. The process of drafting the document was, itself, not without challenges, as members worked systematically to refine the language within each section.

As an observer, I witnessed this process first-hand in Steering Committee meetings. Led by a CE-LHIN representative, the working document would be projected onto a large screen for all members to see. The group would begin with the first section and members would be asked to read it to themselves. The CE-LHIN member would ask for comments on the section shown and members would offer comments or proposed changes. The group would then discuss the proposed change and decide on whether they wanted to accept it, reject it, or make some alteration. The CE-LHIN member would then live-edit the document on a computer and all members could see the changes being made on the overhead projection. This process would be repeated for every section of the document, often returning to previous sections as new comments or suggestions were made. The document would then be e-mailed to all members to review again on their own time following the meeting. At each subsequent meeting this process would be repeated until the guiding framework document was finalized in April 2015.

In the interviews, committee members variously described the process of drafting the document as, "kind of tedious" (SM 7), "a little painful but not too bad" (SM 2), and "not rushed; something that has been tweaked for quite a while" (SM 6). The most commonly-noted challenge in working collaboratively on this process was that it involved, "a lot of collective wordsmithing" (SM 2) which emerged due to the different working vocabularies and acronyms across the health and social housing sectors. As one SM noted, "There's some people that are extremely literal...and are not comfortable unless the language is very, very clear" (SM 4). Despite the repetitive wordsmithing involved, the process of constructing a shared guiding document provided a tool through which members could begin to identify and work through the challenges of their historical and legislative differences, accountability structures, and varied priorities and roles.

> CE-LHIN 2: I'd say the time spent up-front in getting the agreement on guiding principles, and it is a long time, but...it's good time spent. Now we haven't had full fruition of that but I believe that it was good time spent, particularly because these are new partners to one table and we're new. I think we just needed to allow that time. Another learning would be, and again we haven't seen it to fruition but, putting forward a common strategic aim for the group...This is the approach we take and that's an objective, a common goal...a statement we can take out and show people.

It should be noted that the key challenges the group faces are systemic and not easily eradicated through the construction of one document. Rather, the joint framework provided an opportunity to identify the challenges, acknowledge their existence within the context of the group, and allow members an opportunity to begin to address them within their own powers and abilities. In the remainder of this section, I return to the three key challenges and briefly show how members negotiated them within the context of the guiding framework document.

5.1. Legislative and Historical Differences

In Ontario, the LHINs and service managers have emerged within different historical and legislative contexts, resulting in misaligned service boundaries within the province. While a joint document created by the Steering Committee could not change the legislation or retroactively align boundaries, the members could acknowledge these issues and agree to consciously work around them. For instance, a footnote within the document states that a town in one of the service manager counties, "...will be included in planning under this Framework while being beyond the boundary of the Central East LHIN" [60]. Another note within the document states that, "The Central East LHIN will engage directly with the City of Toronto for collaboration and partnership opportunities for residents of Scarborough. When appropriate, opportunities for collaboration and information sharing across all five service managers within the Central East LHIN will be pursued" [60]. This notation is required as Scarborough, part of the City of Toronto, is geographically within the CE-LHIN but is not part of the Steering Committee for reasons beyond the scope of this article.

One concern raised in drafting the document was the inclusion of the word "integration", given the general early resistance to this term when the LHINs first emerged. In the interviews, one CE-LHIN member shared how antipathy toward the term 'integration' impacted the development of the document.

> CE-LHIN 2: ...integration was and is, I would say still, a very foreign term but our municipal partners are more uneasy with the term integration. Similar to how our service providers might have felt in the beginning around the term integration, in understanding it, because we had to spend a lot of time explaining. There was even a suggestion early on at the Steering Committee table that we not use the word integration. We couldn't agree to that but we can define it other ways.

The term integration does appear in the Steering Committee document but, with only one exception, is limited to the name of the LHIN, a description of its mandate, and mention of the Local Health System Integration Act as guiding legislation. The one exception is the inclusion of a continuum of care principle that states, "The LHIN and service managers will work with other key housing, community and health service stakeholders in their communities to ensure services are integrated and provide a continuum of care to meet the varied needs of residents" [60]. While the inclusion of integration in this principle suggests the group has found some consensus to begin to work from, the general lack of the term integration within the document highlights that further work on this issue remains be done.

5.2. Accountability Structures

The members of the Steering Committee each report to an external authority, whether an appointed board, as with the CE-LHIN, or an elected council, as with the service managers. In drafting a joint agreement, the members recognized that they were not only speaking on behalf of those at the table but that they represented the interests of others as well. The challenge associated with the accountability structures was the diversity in that as one SM noted there are, "...differing approval processes and different cultures, and so you're bringing all of those together and it's not easy to get sign-off and language that seems to fit everyone well" (*sic*) (SM 5). The way the Steering Committee attempted to address this challenge in the guiding document was the inclusion of two sections on sponsors and membership accountability.

Sponsors are identified in the document as the Chief Administrative Officers of the Municipality and the Chief Executive Officer of the LHIN or their delegates. These sponsors are there to, "...assist the process as required in obtaining and sustaining support for the process from their respective organizations" [60]. Within the document it further states that sponsors will receive key messages, prepared by the Steering Committee, on a regular basis and following significant events. Under the heading "Membership Accountability", it further states that members will be responsible for liaising with the respective municipal, regional, or provincial leads and organizations, and communicating directly with their sponsors regarding issues, information sharing, and recommendations discussed at the Steering Committee meetings. The final section of the document includes an approval section in which members and their sponsor are required to sign. Although the accountability structures, themselves, have not changed as a result of this framework document, members had the opportunity to explain to one another how their reporting works and to gain a deeper understanding of each other's processes.

5.3. Priorities and Roles

The Steering Committee brings together members from the CE-LHIN, who fund health care services, and representatives from four service manager regions, who fund and administer social housing programs. The differences in priorities and roles is evident in the guiding document, as considerable space is devoted to explicating the purpose of the Steering Committee and the expectations of its members. The document forefronts this information in its first four sections, a representation of the high priority given to clarifying these issues by the Steering Committee members. For instance, the first section entitled "Purpose" states that the group will, "Collaborate during organizational strategic planning with intent to identify common priorities; undertake collaborative service level planning to improve coordination of services and ability for residents to obtain and then retain tenancy; and identify opportunities to align and maximize new investments and existing funding to address needs in [each] community" [60]. Following this section, the document outlines three strategic aims, the Central East LHIN role, and the service manager role.

Creating the guiding document together also allowed members of the Steering Committee to clearly outline what their expectations were and to establish their own limitations as collaborators. The process served as an extended introduction between members. As one CE-LHIN representative stated in an interview, "We did explain where our limitations were around funding and I think that was really helpful...I think really understanding what you can and can't do is incredibly helpful to the process" (CE-LHIN 1). A service manager similarly stated in an interview that, "We're very fortunate to be able to have these discussions...We don't influence the priorities, I don't believe we do, but I believe we influence how the pie gets distributed based on them being more knowledgeable about what some of the pressures we have [are] and what we're trying to do" (SM 4). One example of this sort of influence that emerged out of the framework discussions was an increased allocation of rent supplements within these regions because as one SM noted, "...we were ready and responsive to [CE-LHIN's] questions as they were making their funding decisions" (SM 2).

The different roles of the CE-LHIN as a system wide planner and service managers as municipal planners initially raised concerns that the Steering Committee table, "...doesn't become another place where the loudest voice gets a share of the pie and that it's not just about the LHIN and their money, but it's about the housing piece as well" (SM 4). The Steering Committee recognized this challenge and attempted to address it within the guiding document by including a statement that reads:

> The Steering Committee will adopt a consensus model of decision-making for recommendations/advice. As such, deliberations will seek to build consensus on the most acceptable advice/direction considering the best interests of residents. Where consensus cannot be reached, the Steering Committee will present a summary of the deliberations to their respective Sponsors for input and direction [60].

A footnote within this passage defines consensus as, "general or widespread agreement among all the members of a group" [60]. The consensus model may mean that decisions are not unanimous and some members may be unsatisfied with future decisions. However, a service manager noted, "We're all also pretty reasonable people and so we say as long as there's a rational approach to the allocation of funds, we'll probably all be good with that" (SM 5). This brief discussion of the guiding document is not exhaustive but is meant to demonstrate examples of how members have used the creation of this document to acknowledge and attempt to work through the key challenges they face.

6. Conclusions

Homelessness is a pressing issue in Canada, and other parts of the world, that requires a systems approach. In central east Ontario, a group of service managers and health system planners have formed a collaboration to better coordinate health and housing services for members of their respective communities. This ethnographic study of the group highlighted three key challenges that emerged: historical and legislative differences, varying accountability structures, and different responsibilities and roles. The Steering Committee recognized these challenges and spent a considerable amount of their initial time together drafting a joint guiding framework document that acknowledged these issues and attempted to work through them. The process of jointly creating the principles and terms was described as being just as important as, if not more than, the actual document itself. Working collaboratively on creating the document opened a narrative space at the table for members to deconstruct central aspects of their own work, while learning about those of their partners.

Throughout the interviews, participants clearly identified and reflected on the challenges that emerged through the first year of the Steering Committee. Integrated care remains relatively new in Canada and across North America, with a more developed presence in the United Kingdom [2]. As such, it is foreseeable that issues might arise pertaining to legislative misalignment, differing accountability structures, and a focus on collective *versus* individual interests. Similar challenges have been noted in the UK, related to coordinating health and social care budgets [49,50], characteristics of individuals who assume leadership roles [51], and sharing data freely between collaborators [53]. Homelessness is a prevalent issue in Canada, and studies have shown that combining health and social care has effective outcomes for physical and mental health [37,38], quality of life [39], life satisfaction [40], and the use of emergency health services [41].

The positive outcomes related to integrated care efforts, like supportive housing combined with health and wellness services, lends support to increased investments in combined health and social care for homeless persons. While challenges may be likely to emerge when parties collaborate across sectors, there is also the possibility for innovative practice to emerge. The literature suggests that integrated care is most effective when targeting the highly-intensive service-users [38], when efforts are supported by expertise, multi-service partnerships, and strong leadership [43], and when collaborations are outlined in documents that hold parties accountable to one another [52]. While the members of the central east Ontario Steering Committee continue to navigate the complex relations that underlie their collaborative system planning work, the year together has brought about key learnings that others can adopt and build upon.

The first key learning is that it is possible to bring stakeholders together, even if they have no established pre-existing relationship. The members of the Steering Committee were brought together based on a shared interest in aligning social housing and health supports, despite not having collaborated before. The second lesson is that challenges, while likely to emerge when working intersectorally, are not insurmountable and may even be beneficial in opening a dialogue. Third, members of a group, such as the Steering Committee discussed here, should devote time to identifying their differences and explaining their roles, expectations, abilities, and limitations to one another even if they share similar positions. Fourth, the creation of a joint document, while potentially time consuming, is a valuable exercise that provides a tangible resource for the group members over the duration of the partnership. The joint document produced by this Steering Committee is publicly available as a model [60], although individual groups are strongly encouraged to adapt it to their own work. Finally, participation in a collaborative group that brings different system planners together can be one step toward improving systemic challenges, if not eradicating them altogether.

In this article, I discussed how challenges emerged in relation to the Steering Committee's work and how the members collectively worked to try to overcome them. The creation of a joint document guiding their work provided a process through which members came to better understand and appreciate one another's language, capabilities, and limitations. Integrated care is increasingly becoming recognized as a valuable system planning approach, particularly for addressing the needs of vulnerable individuals. While collaborative approaches like the Steering Committee may pose challenges for members, they also provide the tools for working through them.

Acknowledgments: The research project discussed in this article was funded through a Trent University Canadian Institutes of Health Research Internal Operating Grant (Number 23715 to author). The author would like to thank research assistants Matt Tallon and Amy (Olivia) Sayles, as well as all research participants for their time and contributions to the study. The author would also like to thank three anonymous reviewers for their helpful comments and suggestions.

Conflicts of Interest: The author declares no conflict of interest.

References

1. Nigel Keohane. *A Problem Shared? Essays on the Integration of Health and Social Care*. London: The Social Market Foundation, 2015.
2. Public Health Englan. *Local Leadership, New Approaches: How New Ways of Working Are Helping to Improve the Health of Local Communities*. London: Public Health England, 2015.
3. The Regional Municipality of Durham. *At Home in Durham: Durham Region Housing Plan 2014–2024*. Whitby: The Regional Municipality of Durham, 2013.
4. City of Kawartha Lakes. *Building Strong Communities: Housing and Homelessness Plan 2014–2023*. Lindsay: City of Kawartha Lakes, 2013.
5. Northumberland County. *Northumberland Housing and Homelessness Plan 2014–2023*. Cobourg: Northumberland County, 2013.
6. City of Peterborough. *Peterborough: 10-Year Housing and Homelessness Plan 2014–2024*. Peterborough: City of Peterborough, 2013.
7. Charles J. Frankish, Stephen W. Hwang, and Darryl Quantz. "Homelessness and health in Canada: Research lessons and priorities." *Canadian Journal of Public Health* 96 (2005): S23–29.
8. Stephen W. Hwang. "Homelessness and health." *Canadian Medical Association Journal* 164 (2001): 229–33.
9. Katharine Kelly, and Tullio Caputo. "Health and street/homeless youth." *Journal of Health Psychology* 12 (2007): 726–36.
10. Alistair Story. "Slopes and cliffs in health inequities: Comparative morbidity of housed and homeless people." *The Lancet* 382 (2013): S93.
11. Isolde Daiski. "Perspectives of homeless people on their health and health needs priorities." *Journal of Advanced Nursing* 58 (2007): 273–81.
12. Stephen Hwang, Tim Aubry, Anita Palepu, Susan Farrell, Rosane Nisenbaum, Anita Hubley, Fran Klodawsky, Evie Gogosis, Elizabeth Hay, Shannon Pidlubny, and *et al.* "The health and housing in transition study: A longitudinal study of the health of homeless and vulnerably housed adults in three Canadian cities." *International Journal of Public Health* 56 (2011): 609–23.

13. Kristy Buccieri, and Stephen Gaetz. *Facing FAQs: H1N1 and Homelessness in Toronto*. Toronto: Canadian Observatory on Homelessness, 2015.
14. Stephen W. Hwang, Angela Colantonio, Shirley Chiu, George Tolomiczenko, Alex Kiss, Laura Cowan, Donald A. Redelmeier, and Wendy Levinson. "The effect of traumatic brain injury on the health of homeless people." *Canadian Medical Association Journal* 179 (2008): 779–84.
15. Jane Topolovec-Vranic, Naomi Ennis, Angela Colantonio, Michael D. Cusimano, Stephen W. Hwang, Pia Kontos, Donna Ouchterlony, and Vicky Stergiopoulos. "Traumatic brain injury among people who are homeless: A systematic review." *BMC Public Health* 12 (2012): 1059.
16. Rafael L.F. Figueiredo, Stephen W. Hwang, and Carlos Quiñonez. "Dental health of homeless adults in Toronto, Canada." *Journal of Public Health Dentistry* 73 (2013): 74–78.
17. Stephen Gaetz, Valerie Tarasuk, Naomi Dachner, and Sharon Kirkpatrick. "'Managing' homeless youth in Toronto: Mismanaging food access and nutritional well-being." *Canadian Revue of Social Policy* 58 (2006): 43–61.
18. Valerie Tarasuk, Naomi Dachner, Blake Poland, and Stephen Gaetz. "Food deprivation is integral to the 'hand to mouth' existence of homeless youths in Toronto." *Public Health Nutrition* 12 (2009): 1437–42.
19. Cheryl Forchuk, Rick Csiernik, and Elsabeth Jensen. *Homelessness, Housing, and Mental Health: Finding Truths—Creating Change*. Toronto: Canadian Scholars' Press Inc., 2011.
20. Ami Rokach. "Private lives in public places: Loneliness of the homeless." *Social Indicators Research* 72 (2005): 99–114.
21. Michelle N. Grinman, Shirley Chiu, Donald A. Redelmeier, Wendy Levinson, Alex Kiss, George Tolomiczenko, Laura Cowan, and Stephen W. Hwang. "Drug problems among homeless individuals in Toronto, Canada: Prevalence, drugs of choice, and relation to health status." *BMC Public Health* 94 (2010): 94.
22. Maritt Kirst, Tyler Frederick, and Patricia G. Erickson. "Concurrent mental health and substance use problems among street-involved youth." *International Journal of Mental Health and Addiction* 9 (2011): 543–53.
23. Anne M. Gadermann, Anita M. Hubley, Lara B. Russell, and Anita Palepu. "Subjective health-related quality of life in homeless and vulnerably housed individuals and its relationship with self-reported physical and mental health status." *Social Indicators Research* 116 (2014): 341–52.
24. Chuck K. Wen, Pamela L. Hudak, and Stephen W. Hwang. "Homeless people's perceptions of welcomeness and unwelcomeness in healthcare encounters." *Journal of the Society of General Internal Medicine* 22 (2007): 1011–17.
25. Bernadette Pauly. "Close to the street: Nursing practice with people marginalized by homelessness and substance use." In *Homelessness and Health in Canada*. Edited by Manal Guirguis-Younger, Ryan McNeil and Stephen W. Hwang. Ottawa: University of Ottawa Press, 2014, pp. 211–32.

26. Vanessa Oliver, and Rebecca Cheff. "Sexual health: The role of sexual health services among homeless young women living in Toronto, Canada." *Health Promotion Practice* 13 (2012): 370–77.
27. Kristy Buccieri, and Stephen Gaetz. "Ethical vaccine distribution planning for pandemic influenza: Prioritizing homeless and hard-to-reach populations." *Public Health Ethics* 6 (2013): 185–96.
28. Stephen R. Poulin, Marcella Maguire, Stephen Metraux, and Dennis P. Culhane. "Service use and costs for persons experiencing chronic homelessness in Philadelphia: A population-based study." *Psychiatric Services* 61 (2010): 1093–98.
29. S. Harris Ali. "Tuberculosis, homelessness, and the politics of mobility." *Canadian Journal of Urban Research* 19 (2010): 80–107.
30. Stephen W. Hwang, Alex Kiss, Minnie M. Ho, Cheryl S. Leung, and Adi V. Gundlapalli. "Infectious disease exposures and contact tracing in homeless shelters." *Journal of Health Care for the Poor and Underserved* 19 (2008): 1163–67.
31. Dennis L. Kodner, and Cor Spreeuwenberg. "Integrated care: Meaning, logic, applications, and implications—A discussion paper." *International Journal of Integrated Care* 2 (2002): e12.
32. Deborah K. Padgett, Benjamin J. Henwood, and Sam J. Tsemberis. *Housing First: Ending Homelessness, Transforming Systems and Changing Lives*. New York: Oxford University Press, 2016.
33. Stephen Gaetz, Fiona Scott, and Tanya Gulliver. *Housing First in Canada: Supporting Communities to End Homelessness*. Toronto: Canadian Homelessness Research Network Press, 2013.
34. Paula Goering, Scott Veldhuizen, Aimee Watson, Carol Adair, Brianna Kopp, Eric Latimer, and Tim Aubry. *National Final Report: Cross-Site at Home/Chez Soi Project*. Calgary: Mental Health Commission of Canada, 2014.
35. Suzanne Zerger, Katherine Francombe Pridham, Jeyagobi Jeyaratnam, Stephen W. Hwang, Patricia O'Campo, Jaipreet Kohli, and Vicky Stergiopoulos. "Understanding housing delays and relocations within the Housing First model." *The Journal of Behavioral Health Services & Research* 43 (2016): 38–53.
36. Suzanne Swanton. "Social Housing Wait Lists and the One-Person Household in Ontario." Master's Thesis, University of Waterloo, Waterloo, ON, Canada, 2011.
37. Natalie Waldbrook. "Exploring opportunities for healthy aging among older persons with a history of homelessness in Toronto, Canada." *Social Science & Medicine* 128 (2015): 126–33.
38. Stephen W. Hwang, and Tom Burns. "Health interventions for people who are homeless." *Lancet* 384 (2014): 1541–47.
39. Michelle Patterson, Akm Moniruzzaman, Anita Palepu, Denise Zabkiewicz, Charles J. Frankish, Michael Krausz, and Julian M. Somers. "Housing first improves subjective quality of life among homeless adults with mental illness: 12-Month findings from a randomized control trial in Vancouver, British Columbia." *Social Psychiatry and Psychiatric Epidemiology* 48 (2013): 1245–59.

40. Stephen W. Hwang, Evie Gogosis, Catharine Chambers, James R. Dunn, Jeffrey S. Hoch, and Tim Aubry. "Health status, quality of life, residential stability, substance use, and health care utilization among adults applying to a supportive housing program." *Journal of Urban Health: Bulletin of the New York Academy of Medicine* 88 (2011): 1076–90.
41. Angela Russolillo, Michelle Patterson, Lawrence McCandless, Akm Moniruzzaman, and Julian Somers. "Emergency department utilisation among formerly homeless adults with mental disorders after one year of housing first interventions: A randomised controlled trial." *International Journal of Housing Policy* 14 (2014): 79–97.
42. Maritt Kirst, Suzanne Zerger, Vachan Misir, Stephen Hwang, and Vicky Stergiopoulos. "The impact of a housing first randomized controlled trial on substance use problems among homeless individuals with mental illness." *Drug and Alcohol Dependence* 146 (2015): 24–29.
43. Eric Macnaughton, Ana Stefancic, Geoffrey Nelson, Rachel Caplan, Greg Townley, Tim Aubry, Scott McCullough, Michelle Patterson, Vicky Stergiopoulos, Catherine Vallée, and *et al*. "Implementing housing first across sites and over time: Later fidelity and implementation evaluation of a pan-Canadian multi-site housing first program for homeless people with mental illness." *American Journal of Community Psychology* 55 (2015): 279–91.
44. Jennifer S. Volk, Tim Aubry, Paula Goering, Carol E. Adair, Jino Distasio, Jonathan Jetté, Danielle Nolin, Vicky Stergiopoulos, David L. Streiner, and Sam Tsemberis. "Tenants with additional needs: When housing first does not solve homelessness." *Journal of Mental Health* 3 (2015): 1–7.
45. Ryan McNeil, Manal Guirguis-Younger, Laura B. Dilley, Jeffrey Turnbull, and Stephen W. Hwang. "Learning to account for the social determinants of health affecting homeless persons." *Medical Education* 47 (2013): 485–94.
46. Kelly M. Doran, Elizabeth J. Misa, and Nirav R. Shah. "Housing as healthcare—New York's boundary-crossing experiment." *New England Journal of Medicine* 369 (2013): 2374–77.
47. Rebecca Onie, Paul Farmer, and Heidi Behforouz. "Realigning health with care: Lessons in delivering more with less." *Stanford Social Innovation Review* 10 (2012): 28–35.
48. Carol Wilkins. "Connecting permanent supportive housing to hear care delivery and payment systems: Opportunities and challenges." *American Journal of Psychiatric Rehabilitation* 18 (2015): 65–86.
49. Caroline Abrahams. "Caring for an ageing population." In *A Problem Shared? Essays on the Integration of Health and Social Care*. Edited by Nigel Keohane. London: The Social Market Foundation, 2015, pp. 26–29.
50. Richard Bowden. "Joining up health and care to meet each person's needs—A provider's perspective to being patient-centred." In *A Problem Shared? Essays on the Integration of Health and Social Care*. Edited by Nigel Keohane. London: The Social Market Foundation, 2015, pp. 44–47.

51. Jeremy Hughes. "Apart at the seams: The challenge of integrating dementia care." In *A Problem Shared? Essays on the Integration of Health and Social Care*. Edited by Nigel Keohane. London: The Social Market Foundation, 2015, pp. 21–25.
52. Sir John Oldham. "Collective commissioning." In *A Problem Shared? Essays on the Integration of Health and Social Care*. Edited by Nigel Keohane. London: The Social Market Foundation, 2015, pp. 34–38.
53. Tim Kelsey. "Unleashing the power of people: Why transparency and participation can transform health and care services." In *A Problem Shared? Essays on the Integration of Health and Social Care*. Edited by Nigel Keohane. London: The Social Market Foundation, 2015, pp. 39–43.
54. Dorothy Smith. *Institutional Ethnography: A Sociology for People*. Oxford: AltaMira Press, 2005.
55. Sandra Kirby, Lorraine Greaves, and Colleen Reid. *Experience Research Social Change: Methods beyond the Mainstream*, 2nd ed. Peterborough: Broadview Press, 2006.
56. Ontario. "Local Health System Integration Act 2006 (ON) c. 4." Available online: http://www.ontario.ca/laws/statute/06l04 (accessed on 20 November 2015).
57. Housing Services Corporation. *Canada's Social and Affordable Housing Landscape: A Province-to-Province Overview*. Toronto: Housing Services Corporation, 2014.
58. Government of Ontario. "Social Housing Reform Act 2000 (ON) c. 27." Available online: http://www.ontario.ca/laws/statute/00s27 (accessed on 20 November 2015).
59. Government of Ontario. "Housing Services Act 2011 (ON) c. 6." Available online: http://www.ontario.ca/laws/statute/11h06 (accessed on 20 November 2015).
60. Kristy Buccieri. *Ethnography of the Central East Health, Housing, and Homelessness Steering Committee. Report and Toolkit*. Toronto: Homeless Hub, 2015, pp. 44, 45, 48–50.

U.S. Volunteering in the Aftermath of the Great Recession: Were African Americans a Significant Factor?

Vernon B. Carter and Jerry D. Marx

Abstract: The Great Recession weakened U.S. families' abilities to make charitable gifts. Although African Americans are generally especially hard hit by these types of economic crises, they have a long and distinctive history of volunteerism and mutual assistance. Consequently, the purpose of this study is to examine African American volunteering in nonprofit organizations in the aftermath of the 2008–2009 recession. Specifically, we examined race as well as other factors with the potential to influence volunteering in four categories of organizations: poverty organizations, senior service agencies, social action groups, and religious affiliated organizations. Using the Panel Study of Income Dynamics (PSID) data, this secondary analysis produced significant findings regarding volunteerism among African Americans in these community-based organizations.

Reprinted from *Soc. Sci.* Cite as: Carter, V.B.; Marx, J.D. U.S. Volunteering in the Aftermath of the Great Recession: Were African Americans a Significant Factor? *Soc. Sci.* **2016**, 5, 22.

---

1. Introduction

The Great Recession of 2008–2009 represented the worst economic crisis since the Great Depression. Over 3 million workers in the U.S. lost their jobs in 2008 alone; over 3 million households received home foreclosure notices in that year [1]. This economic crisis, which involved a subprime mortgage scandal, hit new African American and Latino homeowners the hardest [2]. Many small nonprofit human service agencies in communities throughout the United States closed even as the demand for assistance soared. The capability of surviving programs including soup kitchens, community action programs, senior services, and homeless shelters to serve the needy depended considerably on community philanthropy. Yet according to USA Giving 2009, total giving to human services in the U.S. (adjusted for inflation) between 2007 and 2009 dropped by 13.5% [3]. Charitable gifts to most types of nonprofit agencies declined during this period, but the decline in charitable giving to human services was greatest.

The recession weakened U.S. families' abilities to make charitable donations. Although African Americans are generally especially hard hit by these types of economic crises, they have a long and distinctive history of volunteerism and mutual assistance. The term "philanthropy" generally refers to acts or gifts done for humanitarian reasons, and therefore, includes volunteerism as well as charitable gifts. However, social exchange theory maintains that no philanthropic effort is purely altruistic (*i.e.*, a one way exchange) [4]. Rather, like all social exchanges, philanthropy is a two-way exchange motivated by benefits to each party in the exchange—in this case, the giver and receiver. Based on social exchange theory and the African American tradition of mutual assistance, we would expect to see significant efforts by African Americans to contribute their assistance as volunteers to fellow community members negatively impacted by the Great Recession.

1.1. African American Philanthropic History

Much of the private nonprofit sector (such as voluntary health and welfare organizations) that developed in the United States is a result of organized religion [5]. The colonial church provided its impoverished members with essential health and human services. In this way, the church acted as extended family to promote well-being in the community. Over time, American religion became increasingly diverse with multiple denominations. For example, the Puritans, Quakers, Anglicans, Baptists, and Catholics were all influential. These groups further increased the complexity of the U.S. social welfare system by developing their own education, health, and human services. In addition to religious groups, social groups (based on race and ethnicity as well as trade) created mutual aid organizations providing a range of member services. Gradually, these aid networks evolved into a third sector, a private nonprofit or "voluntary" sector, which complemented the government and business sectors in colonial America.

The growth of the nonprofit sector was fueled by new religious movements in the colonies. That is, by the mid-1700s, there was an increasing belief that a charitable life led to salvation. This challenged the Puritan belief in salvation only through the grace of God [5]. Thus, philanthropy became more than a one-way act of kindness; it was a means to salvation—thus benefitting the giver of time and money as well. As a result, poor colonists, including colonists of African descent, were provided a chance at salvation through voluntary acts of kindness.

African American philanthropy, therefore, was also a product of the church and the nonprofit services derived from the church [6]. However, the church was even more influential in African American philanthropic history, because it faced fewer restrictions than other institutions. For example, poor black colonists were often denied assistance in the colonial poorhouse system of public assistance. Later, in the early 1800s, state laws in Virginia, Maryland, and North Carolina banned the formation of charitable societies by African Americans. African American establishments unrelated to the church had to conceal their purpose and activities. To achieve this, in-kind services were frequently offered in place of money. For this reason, in addition to the relative lack of money due to slavery and discrimination, volunteerism plays a central role in African American philanthropic history. One of the most notable examples of early philanthropic African American activity was the participation of African American mutual aid organizations in the Underground Railroad. African American activists voluntarily supplied runaway slaves with food, shelter, and money as they sought freedom [7].

Giving and volunteering were also themes in the empowerment of women—both white and black—in the 1800s [5,8]. Traditionally, U.S. women have contributed to causes that benefited them as women and mothers. Faced with oppression, African American women used philanthropy as a tool to promote equality in addition to fulfilling other basic needs. Perhaps the most well-known example is Harriet Tubman's volunteer work with the Underground Railroad. However, less famous African American women were also engaged in philanthropic activities, including mutual aid organizations and women's clubs. For example, 24 African American women created The Phyllis Wheatley Home Association in 1897 to provide housing for elderly African American women in Detroit, Michigan. A second example is the National Association of Colored Women, an organization that offered employment services, child care, and kindergarten to homeless African Americans [5,7].

This tradition of humanitarianism in the African American community is a tradition often overlooked or ignored by U.S. media. That is, the tradition of volunteerism and mutual assistance by African Americans has sustained their local communities, making them better, healthier places to live. It has enabled African American community members to cope, not only with the home foreclosures and job losses of the Great Recession, but also, with the more recent wave of police shootings of young African American men in several U.S. cities. Media images of this violence in African American neighborhoods need to be countered by the more positive images of neighbors helping neighbors in African American communities.

1.2. Study Objective

This study examines African American volunteering in 2010, the year following the 2008–2009 recession. Specifically, we examined race and other potential factors influencing volunteering in four categories of community-based nonprofit organizations: senior service agencies, social action groups, religious affiliated organizations, and poverty organizations serving those in need of food, shelter, and other basic necessities. The negative impact of the Great Recession on vulnerable seniors and the poor was immediately visible. Social action groups are included in this study, because many often serve and advocate for these vulnerable populations. Furthermore, given the fact that local churches often provide basic services such as food and clothing to the needy in their respective communities, the study also examined volunteering in this fourth category of beneficiary.

2. Research

The body of empirical research on African American volunteerism is limited, and the topic is usually examined in the context of broader studies on philanthropy (*i.e.*, giving and volunteering). Findings regarding the influence of race in these studies have been inconsistent. Hall-Russell and Kasberg surveyed 180 African Americans in the states of Michigan, Ohio and Indiana. The 1997 survey, based on a nonrandom sample, was later continued with 650 African Americans in the same three states using face-to-face and telephone interviews. The research concluded that African Americans tended to value contributions of time more than the contributions of money, and view their philanthropy as a "distinctive tradition" based in kinship and general obligation to the African American community. Study participants also preferred contributing through the church when making formal contributions and favored helping in their local neighborhoods [9].

Hunter, Jones, and Boger surveyed alumni donors of Livingstone College, a historically African American college in North Carolina. No sample size was provided; however donors in the 1999 study ([10], pp. 533–34) tended to be more active on volunteer boards in their communities. They also tended to be female, married with children, employed, and a member of the A.M.E. Zion church (a church affiliated with the college) [10].

In 2000, O'Neill and Roberts published their findings of a survey on giving and volunteering in the state of California, which included an over-sample of minority groups in Alameda County. Using a probability sample, a total of 2406 interviews were done statewide, while 1210 interviews were conducted in Alameda County. This study found no significant differences in giving or volunteering among Whites, African-Americans, Latinos, and Asian/Pacific Islanders. Similar findings were obtained in both the statewide and Alameda samples [11].

Jackson examined the philanthropic motivations of young African Americans, employing focus groups with participants aged 26–32. Two focus groups of "balanced gender" were conducted for two hours with six different people in each session. In a 2001 publication, the researcher concluded that a desire to "uplift the race" through philanthropy is very important to young African-Americans and is reflective of the African-American desire to use philanthropy to promote racial equality and justice. However, a majority of these young study participants did not view the church as a viable way of accomplishing this goal, consequently giving very little of their time and money to the church. That said, these findings should be interpreted cautiously, since this study included a small number of participants [12].

Mesch, Rooney, Chin, and Steinberg in 2002 published the results of a random survey of 885 Indiana households, done through The Public Opinion Laboratory at Indiana University-Purdue University Indianapolis. A little over 13% of the sample classified themselves as a minority including 10.1% African American. Minorities in this sample volunteered on average more hours than did Whites (169 to 126 h annually), yet this difference was not statistically significant. In fact, the survey found no statistically significant differences by race in volunteering or charitable giving [13].

Four years later, in a 2006 study, Mesch, Rooney, Steinberg, and Denton used data from Indiana households again to examine the impact of race, gender, and marital status on patterns of volunteering and charitable giving. In this study, the researchers used a multi-method, multi-group research design. This study also did not find race to be significant; the results did show that single females were 18% more likely to be a volunteer and to volunteer 146 h per year more than single men, ceteris paribus. In addition, the probability of being a volunteer increased with education and income levels [14].

Several studies specifically examining race and volunteerism have been published since the Great Recession. Like the earlier studies, findings regarding the influence of race have been inconsistent though. Farmer and Piotrkowski did a 2009 study on potential differences in civic engagement between African and European American women. The study was a secondary analysis using data from the 2000 Social Capital Benchmark Survey. The study found no significant differences between African and European American women in the extent to which they reported working on community projects and volunteering in their places of worship [15].

Tang, Copeland, and Wexler, in a 2012 publication, surveyed differences in volunteer experience and benefits between older Black and White residents of Pittsburgh. Convenience and purposive sampling produced a sample size of 180 residents aged 60 and over. Black participants were less likely than Whites to volunteer in formal organizations. Yet, once committed, Blacks in the sample contributed more time and perceived more benefits from volunteering than White volunteers [16].

More recently, Gutierrez and Mattis examined volunteerism among 211 African American women in a large urban center in the northeast region (city not identified). Participants in the survey ranged in age from 16 to 83 years of age with a mean of 32.42 years. The 2014 study found that current religious involvement was a positive predictor of volunteer engagement, while age positively predicted the number of hours women volunteer annually [17].

There have been several general studies of volunteerism published since the onset of the Great Recession [18–30]. This research found a wide range of factors other than race correlated with volunteerism. These factors include gender, age, religiosity, home ownership, psychological motivations, fields of employment, income, employment status, marital status, residency, and educational level.

Unlike this study, most of this past empirical research does not focus on the beneficiaries of volunteerism in terms of specific nonprofit categories or populations in need, nor did it produce consistent findings regarding race. This study uses the Panel Study of Income Dynamics (PSID) data to analyze the effects of race and several other independent variables on volunteering by U.S. households to organizations that serve the needy. More specifically, we investigate the following four research questions: Was race a significant factor in volunteering in 2010 for the following types of U.S. nonprofit organizations: (1) religious; (2) poverty relief; (3) senior service; and (4) social change.

3. Methods

3.1. Data

The PSID is a public use dataset produced and distributed by the Institute for Social Research at the University of Michigan in Ann Arbor, MI. Created to help evaluate President Lyndon Johnson's War on Poverty, the PSID is essentially a longitudinal survey that has followed a representative sample of 4800 families and their descendants since 1968. The PSID family and individual files contain data on various demographic characteristics as well as other factors potentially influencing household charitable giving and volunteerism. The current study extracted data from the 2011 Public Use Family file, which included household volunteering activities in 2010—the year in which this data was updated.

Reliability is generally strong in survey research, particularly when standardized questionnaires are used, as in this survey [31]. In addition, the large representative sample allows for inferences regarding minority volunteer behavior in the U.S. However, standardized questionnaires tend to be somewhat superficial, thus limiting validity. Furthermore, this study, like all secondary analysis, is limited by the fact that variable operationalization is confined to the existing measurement instrument and data. As a result, validity is generally not as high as when data are collected directly by the researcher for a specific purpose [31]. In this case, although volunteering with the intent to help the needy typically takes place in the four types of nonprofit organizations of interest in this study, the data do not allow for precise descriptions of volunteer activities within these organizations. In addition, the fact that the PSID dataset is not updated annually prevents a more longitudinal analysis of volunteering in the years immediately before and after the Great Recession.

3.2. Measures

3.2.1. Dependent Variables

Regarding the dependent variables, a questionnaire item asked whether or not the Household Head/Wife volunteered (during 2010) for a specific charitable organization. The specific beneficiary organizations we are exploring in this study are categorized as Religious, Poverty, Senior Services, and Social Change agencies. Further descriptions of the dependent variables are found in Table 1.

Table 1. Dependent Variable descriptions.

Variable Name	Description	Coding
Religious	Person performed a volunteer activity at or through your church, synagogue, or mosque, such as serving on a committee, assisting in worship, teaching, or helping others through programs organized by (your/his) place of worship?	1 = Yes, 0 = No
Poverty	Person performed a volunteer activity through organizations to help people in need, such as working at a soup kitchen, building or repairing a house, or providing other basic necessities?	1 = Yes, 0 = No
Senior	Person performed a volunteer activity through organizations for senior citizens, such as helping at a nursing home or a senior citizens center, providing emotional or social support, visiting, driving, or delivering food?	1 = Yes, 0 = No
Social Change	Person volunteered through organizations to bring about social change, such as civic or community action, working for a political party or advocacy group?	1 = Yes, 0 = No

3.2.2. Independent Variables

The study examined the following independent variables: race, Latino ethnicity; age, number of people and children in household; head of households' marital status, religious preference, retirement, education level, employment status, access to a computer; whether or not household lives in a city; household's income and wealth. Further descriptions of the independent variables are found in Table 2.

Table 2. Independent variable descriptions.

Variable Name	Description	Coding
Age (Head)	Age of head of family	1 = 0/39, 2 = 40/59, 3 = 60/79, 4 = 80/max
Race	Race of the head of the family/Wife's race	1 = White, 2 = African American, 3 = AI/AN, 4 = Asian, 5 = Native Hawaiian
Latino	Spanish descent head of the family	1 = yes, 0 = No
Children	Children in household	1 = Children, 0 = no Children
Household	Number of people in household	1 = Two or less people; 0 = 3 or more people
Religious Head	Head of family expresses a religious preference	1 = yes, 0 = No

Table 2. *Cont.*

Variable Name	Description	Coding
Age (Head)	Age of head of family	1 = 0/39, 2 = 40/59, 3 = 60/79, 4 = 80/max
Race	Race of the head of the family/Wife's race	1 = White, 2 = African American, 3 = AI/AN, 4 = Asian, 5 = Native Hawaiian
Latino	Spanish descent head of the family	1 = yes, 0 = No
Children	Children in household	1 = Children, 0 = no Children
Household	Number of people in household	1 = Two or less people; 0 = 3 or more people
Religious Head	Head of family expresses a religious preference	1 = yes, 0 = No

4. Statistical Analysis

The paper's descriptive analyses use an unweighted cross-sectional sample of all PSID responding households in 2011. The study's multivariate analyses use a weighted (see Heeringa, Berglund, and Khan, 2011 for detailed descriptions of the PSID weights) longitudinal sample consisting of 8970 PSID individuals residing in the households at the time of the interview [32].

Bivariate and multivariate analyses were computed to examine the relationships among variables. Regarding multivariate analyses and more specifically logistic regression analyses, an initial model was created by running logistic regression analyses for each independent variable of interest and volunteer activities for beneficiary organizations of interest: religious, poverty, senior organizations, and social change agencies. The results generated odds ratios, standard errors, p values and confidence intervals. Those variables that were found to have a p values ≤ 0.05 were entered into a multivariate logistic regression analysis to identify those variables that were independently associated with each of the dependent giving variables.

5. Findings

5.1. Sample Characteristics

Our sample consists of 8907 respondents. A subsample of 793 respondents who volunteered were analyzed of whom 56% were White (n = 443); 40% were African-American (n = 316); 4% were other (n = 34). (See Table 3.) A subset of Race was reported as 5% ethnically Latino (n = 39) (all percentages are rounded off).

Table 3. Household characteristics of persons who did volunteer activities for organization in 2011; N = 793 (Unweighted).

Variables	N Yes	N No	% Volunteered	Age Mean/Median	SD
Household Characteristics					
Race/ethnicity *					
White	443	350	55.86	46.92/45	17.32
African American	316	477	39.85	42.59/41	15.07
Other	34	783	4.29	43.82/43	16.53
Latino	39	751	4.94	41.85/39	15.46
Gender					
Male	239	554	30.14		
Female	554	239	69.86		
Religious Head	660	133	83.23		
Retired Head	106	390	21.37	50.17/51.5	16.89
College	614	172	78.12		
Household Characteristics					
Number of persons in household	—	—	—	2.60 (mean)	1.47
Number of children in household	222	571	27.99	0.80 (mean)	1.17
Employed—yes	523	270	65.95		
Computer (Head)	637	155	80.43		
City—resides	258	532	32.66		
Income				64,873/45,883	83,648
min/25,000	264	529	33.29		
25,001/50,000	274	519	34.55		
50,001/100,000	194	599	24.46		
100,001/250,000	54	739	6.81		
250,001/max	7	786	0.88		
Wealth				206,077/22,415	885,400
min/25,000	468	325	59.02		
25,001/100,000	130	663	16.39		
100,001/500,000	126	667	15.89		
500,001/max	69	724	8.70		

* Note: Race/ethnicity variables American Indian/Alaskan Native, Native Hawaiian/Pacific Islander, Other (race/ethnicity), were not analyzed because their numbers were insufficient. Also, the exact percentages may be off because of missing data. It would be too cumbersome to note missing data for every analysis. The authors consider the data to be Missing Completely at Random (MCAR).

The percentage of heads of households who reported being religious was 82% (n = 660). In the sample, 21% of heads of households reported being retired (n = 108). The majority or 78% of the heads of household had attended college (n = 614). The average number of persons living in the household was 3 (SD = 1.48) and the average number of children was 1 (SD = 1.17). The employment rate of household heads was 66% (n = 523); 80% owned a computer (n = 637) and 33% lived in a large metropolitan city (258). The mean income for the head of household was $64,873 (SD = $83,648) and the mean wealth and equity was $206,077 (SD = $885,400).

5.2. Research Question #1: Was Race a Significant Factor in Volunteering in 2010 for U.S. Religious Organizations?

The influence of race as well as the other aforementioned independent variables was tested for possible associations with the dependent variable, the head of the family volunteering for religious organizations, many of which serve people in need (See Table 4). Chi-square results showed the following variables associated with household heads volunteering for religious organizations: being African American, age of household head, head of household reported being religious, city residence, and total household wealth.

Subsequent analysis using multivariate regression showed several of these independent variables to be strongly associated with household volunteering for religious organizations (See Table 5). These associations were being African American, being in the 60 to 79 age group, head of household was religious, and living in a city. The factors in the regression analyses are associated with Americans volunteering for these organizations. The results are in the form of odds ratios (OR). The odds ratio and beta coefficient are interchangeable statistics in a logistic regression. The odds ratio lets the reader know the likelihood that Americans are going to volunteer. A predictor that has an OR equal to 2.0, for example, indicates a person is twice as likely to volunteer. While an OR of 0.55 indicates a person is 45% less likely to volunteer. In this case, household heads who were African American were 1.82 times (OR = 1.82; p = 0.00) as likely to volunteer for such organizations. Household heads aged 60 to 79 were 1.89 times (OR = 1.89; p = 0.00) as likely to volunteer for a religious organization. Not surprisingly, household heads who reported being religious volunteered the most. They were 3.29 times (OR = 3.29; p = 0.00) as likely to volunteer for religious organizations. On the negative side, city dwellers were 25% less likely (OR = 0.75; p = 0.041) to volunteer.

The previously described set of independent variables was also tested for possible associations with the dependent variable, wife of head of household volunteering for religious organizations (See Table 6). Chi-square results showed several independent variables associated with the wife volunteering for religious organizations: age, African American, Latinos, head was religious, head is retired, and number of persons in household.

The results of subsequent multivariate regression analysis showed race, age, and household head religious to be statistically significant predictors of the wife (or as previously discussed, "partner") volunteering for religious organizations (See Table 7). More precisely, wives who were African Americans were 1.72 times (OR = 1.72; p = 0.000) as likely to volunteer in religious organizations; those aged 60 to 79 were almost twice as likely (OR = 1.90; p = 0.001). Furthermore, the wife was more likely to volunteer in religious organizations (OR = 3.58; p = 0.000) if the head of the household reported being religious.

Table 4. Bivariate analysis of independent variables association with household head volunteering (weighted).

Variables	Volunteered Religious			Volunteered Poverty			Volunteered Senior			Volunteered Social		
	%Yes	%No	χ^2	%Yes	%No	χ^2	%Yes	%No	χ^2	%Yes	%No	χ^2
Household Characteristics												
Age years			11.0*			0.89			6.23*			2.74*
0/39	33.02	46.72		41.61	40.76		29.4	42.52		34.93	41.57	
40/59	40.87	38.42		36.46	40.28		38.78	39.55		37.62	39.73	
60/79	22.39	12.6		19.45	15.95		27.05	15.31		25.37	15.73	
80/max	3.72	2.26		2.47	3s.01		4.77	2.61		2.08	2.98	
Race/ethnicity												
White	62.33	67.28	3.16	66.94	64.73	0.47	56.15	66.44	6.13*	65.54	65.12	0.01
African American	32.72	26.04	6.36*	29.05	28.72	0.12	42.76	26.93	16.12*	32.03	28.5	0.71
Latinos	5.51	7.49	1.84	3.58	7.609	5.72*	6.90	6.62	0.02	4.90	6.876	0.73
Religious Head	93.96	79.23	52.18*	84.95	85.61	0.07	89.92	84.85	2.75	82.51	85.81	1.02
Retired Head	15.16	11.54	3.40	10.22	13.96	2.76	21.98	11.83	12.24*	14.23	12.95	0.16
College	72.97	76.21	1.60	77.07	74.1	1.00	74.4	74.89	0.02	83.89	73.66	6.49*
Household Characteristics												
Child	33.10	39.16	2.18	41.77	35.64	1.46	35.72	36.93	0.03	38.04	36.7	0.03
Household	51.93	51.07	0.09	61.19	48.39	14.3*	61.76	49.99	7.39*	59.11	50.44	3.46
Employed	73.56	73.72	0.00	76.55	72.87	1.50	59.32	75.65	18.3*	71.09	73.93	0.49
Computer (Head)	85.96	86.86	0.20	87.21	86.24	0.17	83.09	86.95	1.63	90.38	85.99	2.04
City	25.40	30.77	4.15*	33.03	27.14	3.69*	27.54	28.63	0.07	38.29	27.21	7.01*
Income			2.13			0.28			1.11			1.05
min/25,000	15.53	19.21		17.73	17.51		22.56	16.97		15.28	17.96	
25,001/50,000	24.25	23.43		22.44	24.21		25.62	23.52		20.37	24.09	
50,001/100,000	36.07	31.89		34.9	33.33		30.35	34.12		33.12	33.77	
100,001/250,000	21.42	20.27		19.98	21.02		19.0	21.00		24.67	20.31	
250,001/max	2.74	5.2		4.953	3.919		2.46	4.39		6.56	3.87	
Wealth			3.66*			1.09			0.15			1.85
min/25,000	36.76	44.93		38.74	42.36		41.03	41.53		38.55	41.75	
25,001/100,000	17.4	18.27		16.84	18.25		17.43	17.97		13.7	18.43	
100,001/500,000	28.63	22.75		25.98	24.92		27.25	24.96		26.02	25.18	
500,001/max	17.21	14.04		18.45	14.47		14.29	15.54		21.74	14.64	

Source: Weighted data from the Panel Study of Income Dynamics; * $p < 0.05$.

Table 5. A multivariate analysis predicting Head volunteering in organizations (weighted).

	Volunteered Religious		Volunteered Poverty		Volunteered Senior		Volunteered Social	
Variables	OR (CI)	SE (p)	OR (CI)	SE (p)	OR (CI)	SE (p)	OR (CI)	SE (p)
Household Characteristics								
Age years								
0/39	Reference		-	-	Reference	-	-	-
40/59	1.89 (1.36–2.65)	0.32 (0.00)*	-	-	-	-	-	-
60/79	-	-	-	-	-	-	1.74 (1.10–2.75)	0.41 (0.004)*
80/max	-	-	-	-	-	-	-	-
Race/ethnicity								
White	-	-	-	-	Reference	-	-	-
African American	1.82 (1.36–2.44)	0.27 (0.00)*	-	-	2.12 (1.45–3.10)	0.41 (0.00)*	-	-
Latinos	-	-	0.84 (0.36–1.11)	0.07 (0.042)*	-	-	-	-
Religious Head	3.29 (2.16–5.00)	0.70 (0.00)*	-	-	-	-	-	-
Retired Head	-	-	-	-	-	-	-	-
College	-	-	-	-	-	-	2.05 (1.26–3.34)	0.51 (0.004)*
Household Characteristics								
Child	-	-	-	-	-	-	-	-
Household	-	-	1.51 (1.13–2.03)	0.19 (0.006)*	1.27 (0.83–1.94)	0.27 (0.26)	-	-
Employed	-	-	-	-	0.61 (0.37–0.98)	0.15 (0.04)*	-	-
Computer (Head)	-	-	-	-	-	-	-	-
City	0.75 (0.56–1.53)	0.10 (0.041)*	-	-	-	-	1.71 (1.16–2.51)	0.34 (0.006)*
Income								

Table 5. *Cont.*

Variables	Volunteered Religious		Volunteered Poverty		Volunteered Senior		Volunteered Social	
	OR (CI)	SE (p)	OR (CI)	SE (p)	OR (CI)	SE (p)	OR (CI)	SE (p)
min/25,000	-	-	-	-	-	-	-	-
25,001/50,000	-	-	-	-	-	-	-	-
50,001/100,000	-	-	-	-	-	-	-	-
100,001/250,000	-	-	-	-	-	-	-	-
250,001/max	-	-	-	-	-	-	-	-
Wealth								
min/25,000	-	-	-	-	-	-	-	-
25,001/100,000	-	-	-	-	-	-	-	-
100,001/500,000	-	-	-	-	-	-	-	-
500,001/max	-	-	-	-	-	-	-	-

Source: CI stands for Confidence Interval; Weighted data from the Panel Study of Income Dynamics; * $p < 0.05$; Note: to conserve space the data for the non-statistically significant variables American Indian/Alaskan Native, Native Hawaiian/Pacific Islander, Other (race/ethnicity), college were not shown in table.

Table 6. Bivariate analysis of independent variables association with wife volunteering (weighted).

Variables	Volunteered Religious			Volunteered Poverty			Volunteered Senior			Volunteered Social		
	%Yes	%No	χ^2	%Yes	%No	χ^2	%Yes	%No	χ^2	%Yes	%No	χ^2
Household Characteristics												
Age years			12.51*			0.63			7.41*			1.65
0/39	29.57	42.36		35.23	36.44		19.77	38.46		27.86	37.04	
40/59	44.1	46.56		44.01	45.6		47.75	44.95		45.5	45.28	
60/79	23.98	9.17		17.27	16.15		27.12	14.91		24.5	15.57	
80/max	2.36	1.90		3.49	1.80		5.36	1.67		2.136	2.119	
Race/ethnicity												
White	75.29	79.97	2.57	77.4	77.8	0.01	71.02	78.65	2.85	69.54	78.53	3.10
African American	19.5	12.97	6.34*	18.47	15.58	0.79	27.62	14.54	10.79*	25.02	15.26	4.66*
Latinos	5.6	10.34	6.36*	3.35	9.12	5.60*	4.28	8.54	2.16	0.53	8.764	31.2*
Religious Head	92.47	76.05	40.16*	86.61	83.31	1.00	86.08	83.64	0.38	83.65	83.96	0.00
Retired Head	13.92	9.59	3.74*	15.6	10.78	2.89	20.39	10.52	8.70*	14.68	11.39	0.71
Household Characteristics												
Child	29.15	33.87	2.26	35.86	30.92	0.76	31.97	31.74	0.00	32.38	31.71	0.01
Household	37.68	29.43	6.17*	37.69	32.4	1.55	45.87	31.71	8.14*	42.12	32.55	2.72
Employed	78.61	83.4	3.09	75.26	82.45	4.39*	70.1	82.58	9.33*	77.56	81.44	0.72
Computer (Head)	89.75	92.58	2.03	87.05	92.19	3.94*	85.41	92.01	4.55*	90.03	91.33	0.15
City	22.24	25.67	1.32	26.35	23.4	0.58	18.76	24.66	1.53	24.91	23.87	0.04
			1.50			0.52			0.85			1.36
Income												
min/25,000	4.13	6.14		4.85	5.22		4.25	5.27		2.145	5.447	
25,001/50,000	17.5	13.88		15.1	15.74		21.01	14.9		18.34	15.35	
50,001/100,000	42	39.62		38.71	41.36		40.92	40.84		31.77	41.75	
100,001/250,000	31.45	32.78		32.62	31.96		29.7	32.4		40	31.31	
250,001/max	4.92	7.59		8.72	5.71		4.12	6.58		7.735	6.141	
Wealth			3.66			0.36			1.75			1.84
min/25,000	27.1	34.8		29.27	31.41		23.24	32.06		19.59	32.13	5.35*
25,001/100,000	17.45	16.16		14.98	17.35		15.55	17.08		16.88	16.9	
100,001/500,000	33.89	28.8		33.65	30.68		39.92	30.04	3.96*	36.7	30.7	
500,001/max	21.56	20.24		22.1	20.56		21.29	20.81		26.83	20.27	

Source: Weighted data from the Panel Study of Income Dynamics; * $p < 0.05$.

Table 7. A multivariate analysis predicting wife volunteering in organizations (weighted).

Variables	Volunteered Religious		Volunteered Poverty		Volunteered Senior		Volunteered Social	
	OR (CI)	SE (p)	OR (CI)	SE (p)	OR (CI)	SE (p)	OR (CI)	SE (p)
Household Characteristics								
Age years								
0/39	Reference	-	-	-	Reference	-	-	-
40/59	1.90 (1.26–2.80)	0.38 (0.001) *	-	-	-	-	-	-
60/79	-	-	-	-	-	-	-	-
80/max	-	-	-	-	-	-	-	-
Race/ethnicity								
White								
African American	1.72 (1.29–2.28)	0.25 (0.000) *	-	-	2.41 (1.45–3.99)	0.62 (0.001) *	2.11 (1.13–3.97)	0.68 (0.020) *
Latinos	-	-	-	-	-	-	0.076 (0.02–0.32)	0.05 (0.000) *
Religious Head	3.58 (2.32–5.53)	0.79 (0.00) *	-	-	-	-	-	-
Retired Head	-	-	-	-	-	-	-	-
Household Characteristics								
Child	-	-	-	-	-	-	-	-
Household	-	-	-	-	-	-	-	-
Employed	-	-	-	-	-	-	-	-
Computer (Head)	-	-	-	-	-	-	-	-
City	-	-	-	-	-	-	-	-
Income								
min/25,000	-	-	-	-	-	-	-	-
25,001/50,000	-	-	-	-	-	-	-	-
50,001/100,000	-	-	-	-	-	-	-	-
100,001/250,000	-	-	-	-	-	-	-	-
250,001/max	-	-	-	-	-	-	-	-
Wealth								
min/25,000	-	-	-	-	-	-	0.48 (0.25–0.91)	0.16 (0.025) *
25,001/100,000	-	-	-	-	-	-	-	-
100,001/500,000	-	-	-	-	1.74 (0.26–1.49)	0.40 (0.017) *	-	-
500,001/max	-	-	-	-	-	-	-	-

Source: Weighted data from the Panel Study of Income Dynamics; * $p < 0.05$.

5.3. Research Question #2: Was Race a Significant Factor in Volunteering in 2010 for U.S. Poverty Organizations?

The set of independent variables was also tested for possible associations with the dependent variable, head of household volunteering for poverty organizations, which serve people in need of basic necessities like food, shelter, and basic health care (See Table 4). Chi-square analyses show that three variables were significantly associated with head of household volunteering for poverty organizations: being Latino, number of persons in household, and living in a city.

The multivariate regression showed that two variables were significantly associated with the household head volunteering for poverty organizations (See Table 5). Household heads who were Latino were 16% less likely to volunteer for poverty organizations (OR = 0.84, p = 0.042), while heads of larger households were one and a half times more likely to volunteer (OR = 1.51, p = 0.006).

This study also tested for possible associations with the dependent variable, wife of head of household volunteering for poverty organizations (See Table 6). Chi-square results showed three independent variables associated with the wife volunteering for poverty organizations. These variables were Latinos, employed, and head owns a computer.

Subsequent multivariate regression analysis, however, showed none of the independent variables to be a statistically significant predictor of a wife volunteering for poverty organizations (See Table 7). The aforementioned variables came close to statistical significance but all possessed negative associations. The variables Latinos, employed, and the head of household owning a computer decreased the likelihood the wife would volunteer for a poverty agency.

5.4. Research Question #3: Was Race a Significant Factor in Volunteering in 2010 for U.S. Senior Organizations?

Many senior citizens, because of their unemployed status and frail health, suffer from poverty. Because of this vulnerability, race and the other previously described independent variables were also tested for possible associations with the dependent variable, head of household volunteering for senior organizations, many of which serve senior citizens in need of necessities like food and basic health care (See Table 4). Chi-square results showed several independent variables associated with volunteering for senior organizations. These variables were race of household head as well as age, head is retired, employed, and number of persons in household.

Subsequent multivariate regressions showed two of these independent variables to be significant predictors of head of household volunteering for senior service organizations: being African American, and employed (See Table 5). African Americans (OR = 2.12; p = 0.000) were roughly twice as likely to volunteer in senior service organizations. In contrast, household heads who were employed were 39% less (OR = 0.61; p = 0.04) likely to volunteer in these agencies.

The wife's volunteering for senior organizations was examined (See Table 6). Chi-square results showed several independent variables associated with wife volunteering for senior organizations. These variables were race, age, head of household was retired and owned a computer, number of persons in household, and employed.

Subsequent analyses showed two independent variables to be statistically significant predictors of the wife volunteering for senior organizations (see Table 7). These were African American, and wealth. That is, wives who were African American were almost two and half (OR = 2.41; p = 0.001) times more likely to volunteer in senior service organizations. In addition, household wealth being in the \$100,001/\$500,000 bracket (OR = 1.74; p = 0.017) positively influenced the likelihood of the wife volunteering by over one and half times.

5.5. Research Question #4: Was Race a Significant Factor in Volunteering in 2010 for U.S. Social Change Organizations?

The fourth research question explored head of household volunteering for social change organizations, many of which advocate for people in need (See Table 4). Chi-square results showed three independent variables associated with the household head volunteering for social change organizations. These variables were age, attended college, and city.

The results of subsequent multivariate regression analyses showed the same three independent variables to be significant predictors of the household head volunteering for social change organizations (see Table 5). More precisely, those head of households who lived in a city (OR = 1.71; p = 0.006) were more than one and half times likely to volunteer in social change agencies. Household heads aged 60 to 79 (OR = 1.74; p = 0.004) and those who had attended college (OR = 2.05; p = 0.004) were approximately twice as likely to volunteer. Race was not a significant predictor of the household head volunteering for social change organizations.

The list of independent variables was also tested for possible associations with the dependent variable, wife of head of household volunteering for social change organizations (See Table 6). Chi-square results indicated three independent variables associated with the wife volunteering for senior organizations. These variables were African American, Latinos and wealth.

Subsequent multivariate regression analysis showed the same variables to be statistically significant predictors of the wife volunteering for social change organizations (see Table 7). The least likely to volunteer were Latinos. Compared to non-Latinos, they were 92% less like to volunteer (OR = 0.08; p = 0.000). Those with a household wealth in the category of "min/\$25,000" were 52% less likely (OR = 0.48;

$p = 0.025$) to volunteer. However, African American wives were twice (OR = 2.11; $p = 0.020$) as likely to volunteer in social change agencies.

6. Discussion

Our study results indicate that African Americans were significantly active in volunteering for nonprofit organizations that typically help groups most vulnerable to the negative impact of recessions. Historically, those most susceptible in the U.S. have been poor and frail minorities [5]. The Great Recession and its accompanying home foreclosure crisis was no exception, particularly targeting African Americans (as well as Latinos). More specifically, our analysis indicated that being an African American head of a household was a significant factor in that person volunteering for religious organizations—many of which serve people in need. In fact, household heads who were African American were 1.82 times (OR = 1.82; $p = 0.00$) more likely to volunteer for religious organizations than other household heads in this study population (see Table 5). Similarly, multivariate regressions showed that being an African American head of a household was a significant predictor of the head of household volunteering for senior organizations (See Table 5). In this study, heads of households who were African Americans were over twice as likely (OR = 2.12; $p = 0.00$) to volunteer to help seniors in their communities.

These results support earlier empirical research on African American philanthropy in general—that is, encompassing both contributions of cash and time. For example, the 1997 survey by Hall-Russell and Kasberg of 830 African Americans found that African Americans prefer making formal donations of money through the church when they do give, but generally value contributions of time more than cash donations [9]. The survey also found that African Americans view their philanthropy as distinctive with a greater emphasis on personal relationships and "kinship", in the sense that all African Americans are viewed as brothers and sisters.

When our analysis focused just on the wives/partners of household heads, the results were similar. Multivariate regression results indicated that being African American was a significant factor in the wife volunteering for religious organizations (See Table 7). More precisely, wives who were African American were 1.72 times (OR = 1.72; $p = 0.00$) as likely to volunteer for religious organizations. Comparable results were obtained in the analysis of senior organizations (see Table 7). African American wives were almost two and half (OR = 2.41; $p = 0.001$) times more likely to volunteer to assist people in senior organizations than other wives. Furthermore, African American wives were also significantly active in helping others through volunteering in social change organizations. Regression analysis findings (see Table 7) indicated that wives who were African American were over twice as likely (OR = 2.11; $p = 0.020$) to volunteer their time in social change organizations.

This study's use of the PSID and its large representative sample allows for inferences regarding minority volunteer behavior. Yet, like all secondary analysis, this analysis is limited in that our variable operationalization is confined to the existing survey questions. As a result, although volunteering to assist the needy typically occurs in the four types of nonprofit organizations examined in this study, the questionnaire and related data do not allow for more precise descriptions of volunteer activities within these settings.

7. Conclusions

The results of this study are consistent with historical literature on African American philanthropy [5]. In times of crisis, African Americans have typically offered assistance through any number of voluntary acts of kindness. Whether the crisis was escape from slavery, surviving the Great Depression, breaking the bonds of segregation during the Civil Rights Movement, or coping with massive home foreclosure and unemployment in the Great Recession, African Americans made significant voluntary efforts to assist others in their communities. In contrast to media images of violence, hate, and hopelessness in African American communities, such "hands-on" philanthropy furthers trust, collaboration, and empowerment among participants, thereby building social capital and generally healthier communities [33]. Given this, philanthropy and those who practice it play a central role in the health of communities. Our findings indicate that African Americans represent a potentially valuable resource for nonprofit community services dependent on volunteerism. Future research on factors contributing to healthy, sustainable communities should further examine the role of philanthropic factors such as volunteerism, mutual assistance, and financial donations. Given the limitations of this study, such research should also incorporate qualitative data collection methods to offer a more detailed, in-depth examination of voluntary behavior in community nonprofit organizations.

Acknowledgments: The authors would like to acknowledge the research assistance of Rebecca Cole, and undergraduate student, Crystal Napoli.

Author Contributions: Vernon B. Carter and Jerry D. Marx conceived and designed this study; Marx conducted a review of the historical literature on African American philanthropy as well as a review of past empirical research on African American volunteerism; Carter did the statistical analysis and table construction; Carter and Marx shared equally in the writing of the manuscript.

Conflicts of Interest: The authors declare no conflict of interest.

References

1. Kanto, Jodi. *The Obamas*. New York: Little, Brown, and Company, 2012.

2. Salomon, Larry R., Julie Quiroz, Maggie Potapchuk, and Lori Villarosa. "Timeline of Race, Racism, Resistance and Philanthropy 1992–2014." *Critical Issues Forum, Moving Forward on Racial Justice Philanthropy* 5 (2014): 8–22.
3. Center on Philanthropy at Indiana University. *Giving USA 2010: The Annual Report on Philanthropy for the Year 2009. Executive Summary*. Glenview: Giving USA Foundation, 2010, p. 14.
4. Blau, Peter Michael. *Exchange and Power in Social Life*. Piscataway: Transaction Publishers, 1986.
5. Marx, Jerry D. *Social Welfare: The American Partnership*. Boston: Allyn & Bacon, 2004, pp. 47–49.
6. Jansson, Bruce S. *The Reluctant Welfare State: American Social Welfare Policies—Past, Present, and Future*. Belmont: Thomson Brooks/Cole, 2005.
7. Carter, Vernon B., and Jerry Marx. "What motivates African-American charitable giving: Findings from a national sample." *Administration in Social Work* 31 (2007): 67–85.
8. Marx, Jerry D. "Women and human services giving." *Social Work* 45 (2000): 27–38.
9. Hall-Russell, Cheryl, and Robert H. Kasburg. *African-American Traditions of Giving and Serving*. Indianapolis: Indiana University Center on Philanthropy, 1997.
10. Hunter, Catrelia S., Enid B. Jones, and Charlotte Boger. "A study of the relationship between alumni giving and selected characteristics of alumni donors of Livingstone College, NC." *Journal of Black Studies* 29 (1999): 524–39.
11. O'Neill, Michael, and William L. Roberts. *Giving and Volunteering in California*. San Francisco: Institute for Nonprofit Organization Management, 2000, pp. 51–68.
12. Jackson, Tysus D. "Young African Americans: A new generation of giving behaviour." *International Journal of Nonprofit and Voluntary Sector Marketing* 6 (2001): 243–53.
13. Mesch, Debra J., Patrick Michael Rooney, William Chin, and Kathryn S. Steinberg. "Race and gender differences in philanthropy: Indiana as a test case." *New Directions for Philanthropic Fundraising* 37 (2002): 65–77.
14. Mesch, Debra J., Patrick Michael Rooney, Kathryn S. Steinberg, and Brian Denton. "The effects of race, gender, and marital status on giving and volunteering in Indiana." *Nonprofit & Voluntary Sector Quarterly* 35 (2006): 565–87.
15. Farmer, G. Lawrence, and Chaya S. Piotrkowski. "African and European American Women's Volunteerism and Activism: Similarities in Volunteering and Differences in Activism." *Journal of Human Behavior in the Social Environment* 19 (2009): 196–212.
16. Tang, Fengyan, Valire Carr Copeland, and Sandra Wexler. "Racial differences in volunteer engagement by older adults: An empowerment perspective." *Social Work Research* 36 (2012): 89–100.
17. Gutierrez, Ian A., and Jacqueline S. Mattis. "Factors predicting volunteer engagement among urban-residing African American women." *Journal of Black Studies* 45 (2014): 599–619.
18. Marta, Elena, and Maura Pozzi. "Young People and Volunteerism: A Model for Sustained Volunteerism during the Transition to Adulthood." *Journal of Adult Development* 15 (2008): 35–46.

19. Scharffs, Brett G. "Volunteerism, Charitable Giving, and Religion: The U.S. Example." *Review of Faith and International Affairs* 7 (2009): 61–67.
20. Rotolo, Thomas, John Wilson, and Mary Elizabeth Hughes. "Homeownership and Volunteering: An Alternative Approach to Studying Social Inequality and Civic Engagement." *Sociological Forum* 23 (2010): 570–87.
21. Einolf, Christopher J. "Gender Differences in the Correlates of Volunteerism and Charitable Giving." *Nonprofit and Voluntary Sector Quarterly* 40 (2011): 1092–112.
22. Nesbit, Rebecca, and Beth Gazley. "Patterns of Volunteer Activity in Professional Associations and Societies." *International Society for Third-Sector Research* 23 (2012): 558–83.
23. Lim, Chaeyoon, and Carol Ann MacGregor. "Religion and Volunteering in Context: Disentangling the Contextual Effects of Religion on Voluntary Behavior." *American Sociological Review* 77 (2012): 747–79.
24. Choi, Namkee G., and Diana M. DiNitto. "Predictors of Time Volunteering, Religious Giving, and Secular Giving: Implications for Non-Profit Organizations." *Journal of Sociology and Social Welfare* 39 (2012): 93–120.
25. Forbes, Kevin F., and Ernest M. Zampelli. "Volunteerism: The Influences of Social, Religious, and Human Capital." *Nonprofit and Voluntary Sector Quarterly* 43 (2012): 227–53.
26. Bidee, J., T. Vantilborgh, R. Pepermans, G. Huybrechts, J. Willems, M. Jegers, and J. Hofmans. "Autonomous Motivation Stimulates Volunteers' Work Effort: A Self-Determination Theory Approach to Volunteering." *International Society for Third-Sector Research* 24 (2013): 32–47.
27. Paxton, Pamela, Nicholas E. Reith, and Jennifer L. Glanville. "Volunteering and the Dimensions of Religiosity: A Cross-National Analysis." *Review of Religious Research* 56 (2014): 597–625.
28. Einolf, Christopher J., and Deborah Philbrick. "Generous or Greedy Marriage? A Longitudinal Study of Volunteering and Charitable Giving." *Journal of Marriage and Family* 76 (2014): 573–86.
29. Lancee, Bram, and Jonas Radl. "Volunteering over the Life Course." *Social Forces* 93 (2014): 833–62.
30. Whitehead, George I., III. "Correlates of Volunteerism and Charitable Giving in the Fifty States." *North American Journal of Psychology* 16 (2014): 531–36.
31. Rubin, Allen, and Earl Babbie. *Research Methods for Social Work*, 2nd ed. Pacific Grove: Brooks/Cole, 1993.
32. Heeringa, Steven G., Patricia A. Berglund, Katherine Mcgonagle, and Robert Schoeni. "Panel Study of Income Dynamics. Construction and Evaluation of the Longitudinal Individual and Family Weights." In *Panel Study of Income Dynamics Technical Report*. Ann Arbor: Survey Research Center, 2011.
33. Roseland, Mark. *Toward Sustainable Communities*. Gabriola Island: New Society, 2012.

Intersectoral Mobilization in Child Development: An Outcome Assessment of the Survey of the School Readiness of Montreal Children

Isabelle Laurin, Angèle Bilodeau, Nadia Giguère and Louise Potvin

Abstract: In 2006, the department of public health in Montreal, Quebec, Canada, conducted the *Survey of the School Readiness of Montreal Children*. After unveiling the results in February 2008, it launched an appeal for intersectoral mobilization. This article documents the chain of events in the collective decision-making process that fostered ownership of the survey results and involvement in action. It also documents the impacts of those findings on intersectoral action and the organization of early childhood services four years later. The results show that the survey served as a catalyst for intersectoral action as reflected in the increased size and strength of the actor network and the formalization of the highly-anticipated collaboration between school and early childhood networks. Actors have made abundant use of survey results in planning and justifying the continuation of projects or implementation of new ones. A notable outcome, in all territories, has been the development of both transition-to-kindergarten tools and literacy activities. The portrait drawn by the research raises significant issues for public planning while serving as a reminder of the importance of intersectoral mobilization in providing support for multiple trajectories of child preschool development.

Reprinted from *Soc. Sci.* Cite as: Laurin, I.; Bilodeau, A.; Giguère, N.; Potvin, L. Intersectoral Mobilization in Child Development: An Outcome Assessment of the Survey of the School Readiness of Montreal Children. *Soc. Sci.* **2015**, *4*, 1316–1334.

1. Introduction

The importance of providing support for child development during the first years of life has been abundantly reinforced over the past two decades [1–3]. All children do not start out in life with the same opportunities or the same social capital [4–6]. Poverty places some children in contexts that prevent them from developing at the same rate as others, and this reality becomes apparent when they start school [7–9]. The differences observed in children constitute a form of inequality that can be reduced by intelligent public policies that support families in precarious socio economic situations [4,10].

To obtain a better understanding of the spheres of development necessitating preventative action, researchers developed the Early Development Instrument (EDI), a population measure of child development [11]. The tool, developed in Ontario during the 1990s, is now used throughout Canada and other countries to evaluate children's levels of development when they start school. It is also designed to serve as a planning tool for mobilizing networks of stakeholders to effect transformations in living conditions, resources and services [12].

In the wake of the pan-Canadian movement for child development, the department of public health of the Montreal Health and Social Services Agency in the province of Quebec, Canada, launched the *Montreal Summit Initiative on School Readiness* in 2008, as a follow-up to its *Survey of the School Readiness of Montreal Children* [13,14]. The survey used the EDI, and revealed that 35% of Montreal children were vulnerable in at least one developmental area when they started school. It found considerable differences between Montreal neighbourhoods, with results ranging from 23% to 43% [15]. The objective of the *Summit Initiative* was to identify child-development related needs on the Island of Montreal and to improve service provision by mobilizing intersectoral partners concerned with early childhood services at the local level of 12 Health and Social Services Centres[1] (HSSC) as well as on a regional level. The initiative also fell under the broader objectives of Quebec's provincial public health program for 2003–2012 [16], which, following the World Health Organization's example, made community development one of the province's key public health intervention strategies for promoting health and reducing social inequalities in health [17]. Despite the popularity of this type of community-level intervention, little research has been done on the processes involved in those interventions. Consequently, there is underproduction of theoretical knowledge and underuse of those practices [18,19].

To offset the situation, this article presents the collective decision-making process used during the *Montreal Summit Initiative on School Readiness* to transform early-childhood service organization in Montreal. The article also documents processes of change in early childhood service organization and actor mobilization after EDI data were released. Although many mobilization initiatives have been carried out in Canada since the early 2000s [20–22], no study has documented the impact of these surveys on collective planning in communities. A survey of nine Canadian provinces was conducted [23], but it presents general observations and not processes that lead to changes in communities. The study by Laurin *et al.* is informative in this regard; however the scope of those results is limited since the study focused on only one Montreal neighbourhood [18].

---

[1] In Quebec, Health and Social Services Centres are public organizations that provide front-line health and social assistance services, such as home care for elderly or disabled persons, prenatal classes and early childhood services. Each of the 12 HSSC's in Montreal is associated with a specific territory that determines the population it serves.

The current study was undertaken to document the processes by which the *Survey of the School Readiness of Montreal Children* fostered actor mobilization in all districts of Montreal. This article documents (1) the chain of events in the collective decision-making process that fostered ownership of the survey results and actor mobilization; and (2) the ongoing effects on intersectoral action and service organization throughout Montreal four years later.

2. Methods

2.1. Theoretical Framework

Actor-network theory (ANT), a social theory concerned with how actions by networks of actors are constituted and operate, provided the general framework for analysis of the population health initiatives arising out of the *Summit Initiative* intersectoral action and community mobilization. This theory is recognized as being a conceptually useful tool for appraising complex situations and analysing the production of change [19]. ANT perceives such initiatives as complex systems of action, *i.e.*, socio-technical networks (STN), which generate social reproduction/transformation processes in achieving certain end goals [19,24]. These process-generating networks are described as socio-technical due to their mobilization of social actors, knowledge (both scientific and experiential), and goods [25–27]. Social actors in such networks are characterized by their social position, identity, interests, and the issues that mobilize them in the situation under study. Setting up action networks requires constant translation that consists in generating clear, meaningful links toward action among heterogeneous entities involved in a situation [28]. The general purpose of such systems of action is the orientation of social transformations at their level, and the response to situations deemed problematic.

In such networks of multi-sectoral actors, decisions are not the product of a single actor or of a response to an isolated situation, but rather of a process shaped by the actions and interactions of influential actors, both inside and outside a system of action, within a specific context. Out of these actions and interactions arise different events (what happens) that constitute the relevant data for the study of such processes. The decision-making process is thus comprised of a chain of events out of which the decision is built [24,29]. When public institutions play a role in these decision-making processes (e.g., as financial backers), the primary *modus operandi* used by these actor networks to construct decisions remains programmed action (planning, implementation, sustainability and reflexivity), exercised pragmatically in light of the different perspectives and interests involved [30,31]. In such systems, programmed action is necessarily a process that occurs at a specific time and place and in a specific context. It is a dynamic entity that both transforms and is transformed by this context. Its means of action are the creation, reconfiguration and extension of the socio-technical network that allows for the input of actors, goods, and new knowledge.

2.2. Design

The research design was a three-year multiple-case study [32] monitoring the activities of the regional committee and six local committees during both the Montreal Summits phase (February 2008–May 2009), and the post-summit phase (June 2009 until the end of research in December 2011). The systems of action (actor networks and interventions) mobilized around the issue of school readiness constituted the principal unit of analysis. This is an interpretive study in that data are interpreted in light of the theoretical framework described earlier. The study looks at processes and their outputs as they occurred *in situ*, beyond the researchers' control.

2.3. Participants

The study focuses on one regional and six local systems of action selected from among the 12 HSSCs in Montreal, based on two criteria: (1) having a high percentage and number of vulnerable children in terms of school readiness, based on survey data; and (2) ensuring regional representation. Sociodemographic representation of the six districts reflects a wide range of situations: some are very ethnically diverse, some are very poor, and some comprise large zones of poverty even though they are considered middle-income areas. The regional and local systems of action comprise intersectoral actors involved in preparing children for school.

2.4. Data Sources and Collection Methods

One community organizer from each of the six districts under study, together with one representative from the regional committee were asked and agreed to participate as research partners. They passed on to the research team all administrative documentation relevant to the project. Three methods of data collection were used: (1) note-taking during non-participant direct observation of regional events and meetings of both regional ($n = 9$) and local ($n = 24$) committees; (2) document analysis of the minutes of the meetings of regional and local summit organizing and monitoring committees ($n = 24$) as well as of other local early childhood collaborative bodies ($n = 140$), and of administrative and planning documents ($n = 271$); (3) semi-structured individual and small group (2 to 3 people) interviews, as a complement to the analysis of administrative documentation, conducted one ($n = 38$), and two ($n = 24$) years later. At the regional level, semi-structured individual interviews were carried out with 14 committee members from the health, education, daycare, community, municipal, charitable and immigration sectors. At the local level, semi-structured interviews were conducted with each of the community organizers from the six territories, accompanied by one or more representatives from other sectors in accordance with the organizer's wishes.

2.5. Analysis

Data processing consisted of the production of a database comprised of pertinent excerpts from the administrative documents, interviews, and observation field notes, coded according to the study's theoretical framework. Two matrices were used to organize and analyze data. The first describes the composition of socio-technical networks—organizational actors (e.g., HSSC, schools, and daycares) and collective actors (e.g., committees), mobilized goods and knowledge. The second classifies decision-making events by programmed action: planning, implementation, sustainability and reflexivity. Data were organized chronologically to reconstruct *a posteriori* the principal chain of events constituting the collective process of programmed action. Triangulation of data from the various sources was used to ensure the validity of results.

The analysis focused on identifying the actor networks involved in the *Summit Initiative*, the knowledge and goods or resources they mobilized, and the role played by survey data. A second focus was the chain of events composing the summit and post-summit decision-making processes that showed how choices were made and decisions taken, and the outcomes on services described by the actors.

The results were validated at a sharing activity in April 2011 during which regional actors or those involved in the six local cases discussed the results for the 2008–2009 period that had ended with a regional summit. For the post-summit period (2009–2011), result validation and sharing activities were not possible due to the very large number of local actors in the various sectors involved. Rather, we opted to validate survey data, established with administrative sources and observation, through interviews with the actors concerned. Triangulation of documentary sources and observation led us to retain, in the matrices, data that could not be validated in interviews, even though administrative documents demonstrated the existence of those survey data.

3. Results

The appeal for action made by the department of public health of the Montreal Health and Social Services Agency (DPH) following the release of the survey data led to the extension and consolidation of actor networks involved in early childhood issues, both regionally and locally. These networks of actors took ownership of the survey data, planning and implementing actions they judged pertinent and feasible. Two important collective decisions were characteristic of this process. First, at the end of the 15-month summit phase, regional and local actors collectively managed to transform child school readiness into an important social issue and called for mobilization for action. Second, during the post-summit period, local solutions were structured around the idea that child development issues or problems of school readiness could be reduced through the increased availability and accessibility of services for vulnerable children in the community. The following analysis presents the chain of key events and the actors involved in elaborating these decisions.

3.1. The Collective Decision-Making Process during the Summits: The Transformation of Survey Results into an Important Social Issue

A series of seven sequential and occasionally overlapping events provided the framework for the decision-making process during the summit phase. It is important to note that while preparing the Survey of the School Readiness of Montreal Children to be conducted in 2006, the survey's instigators met with the principal early childhood actors in the 12 HSSC territories to inform them of the survey objectives and the proposed mobilization approach. This tour also served as an opportunity to consult communities on the establishment of territorial divisions smaller than HSSC territories, more representative of actual living environments, and more useful from an intervention perspective.

Table 1 presents information on the *Survey of the School Readiness of Montreal Children* and the *Montreal Summit Initiative on School Readiness* (2005–2008) that chronologically lists some of the events that ensued.

3.1.1. Publication of Survey Results—February 2008

In February 2008, the DPH published the results of the Survey of the School Readiness of Montreal Children. Given the finding that 35% of Montreal children were vulnerable in at least one developmental area when they started school, it was stated that the time of "one-size-fits-all" solutions was past, and that it was important to look at what was working locally and to fine-tune the interventions. Concurrently, it appealed for cooperation among the various actors concerned with preparing children for school (health, education, and daycare services networks, community groups, the City and philanthropic groups). It was at this moment that the Summit Initiative was announced. The Initiative would use Montreal's public health infrastructure comprised of the DPH and the 12 HSSC, which would assume responsibility for implementing the initiative at the local level from February 2008 to May 2009. At the end of the 12 local summits—one per HSSC territory— and to conclude the process, a regional event would be held to which all Montreal early childhood actors would be invited.

Table 1. Montreal Summit initiative on School Readiness.

	Stakeholders involved	Accomplishments	Important dates
Survey en route pour l'école !	A survey conducted by the DPH Partners: Lucie and André Chagnon Foundation • The 5 Montreal school boards • Research unit on children's psychosocial maladjustment (GRIP) • Centre 1,2, 3 Go! • Social Development Canada	• Met with school boards to enlist their collaboration in collecting data. • Met with the main early childhood stakeholders in each of Montreal's 12 HSSC to inform them of the survey objectives and of mobilization efforts • Defined the new divisions in Montreal (more significant for communities) into 101 neighbourhoods • Collected data from educators • Produced and released a series of reports that present a portrait of the school readiness of Montreal children using the Early Development Instrument (EDI) to measure the five domains of readiness	2005 February 2006 February 2008
Local summits	Led by: the 12 HSSC, in collaboration with: local partners Support from: DPH	• Organized and carried out 12 local summits (1 per HSSC territory), each of which reached over 100 people • Fruitful exchanges that fostered a shared interpretation of the situation, leading to identification of a number of challenges and avenues for solutions regarding resource development, service organization and ways to work with children and families • Wrote 12 synthesis reports on discussions held during the summits (with the help of notes taken by the DPH during various activities) • Defined three action priorities for each territory	Fall 2008 to Spring 2009
Montreal Summit	Comité régional pour une action concertée en développement de l'enfant	• Organized and carried out two theme days (the role of parents and distinctive characteristics of Montreal) that brought to the fore specific issues prior to the local summits • Conducted iterative analyses of information emerging from local summits to ensure the Montreal Summit is in line with local concerns • Carried out the Montreal Summit • Promoted the three priorities established by the HSSC and their partners	2008–2009 28/05/2009
Overview of the process	DPH	• Disseminated a synthesis document outlining the main concerns expressed by a majority of partners throughout the summits initiative • Disseminated a video of the highlights of the Montreal Summit on school readiness (28 May 2009)	Summer 2009

3.1.2. Involvement of Regional Intersectoral Partners in the Summit Process—March 2008

In March 2008, the DPH called on its regional partners to join it in the summit process. A regional intersectoral collaborative body (RIC) was created bringing together partners from the health care network, education, daycare, community and charitable organizations, and from the Ministry of Immigration. City of Montreal officials (from the library network and the social development sector) asked to be included in order to participate in the collective discussion, as they considered themselves as having an informal educator role in early childhood support. The RIC's mandate included support for the summit process as well as ownership of the survey data. This included reflecting on the issues raised by the researchers in their report, that is, accessibility and quality of childcare services and kindergarten for four-year-olds; the capacity of public policies and programs to lift families out of poverty and reduce social inequalities; and convergent and complementary actions.

3.1.3. Act 7 and the Creation of the Fund for Early Childhood Development—March 2008

In March 2008, only a few brief weeks after the survey results had been released, the Government of Quebec announced in its budget the introduction of Bill 7, creating the *Fund for Early Childhood Development* in partnership with a private foundation. The fund, for which one of the justifications was the survey results, was intended to inject CAD$400 million over 10 years into local initiatives targeting children aged five and under living in poverty. The Government of Quebec then launched a public hearing in which 19 organizations took part. The Government concluded that most organizations agreed with the fund. However, a press release was immediately issued by a federation of family associations rectifying the Government's conclusions and stating that only seven organizations stood in support of the fund, while eight groups were calling for either a moratorium on the bill or its withdrawal. The bill was nevertheless adopted in the fall of 2009, and the public-philanthropic partnership launched its activities in the spring of 2010.

3.1.4. Theme Days and Discussions in Preparation for the Summits—2008–2009

Other issues in addition to the ones submitted to actors by the RIC in the survey report emerged as a result of the mobilization, and were initially explored by the RIC in preparatory discussions for the summits. The RIC organized two theme days, one devoted to the role of parents in service development, and the other to ethnic diversity, population mobility, and poverty—unique Montreal concerns. In the actors' opinion, it was vital that discussions of the provision of services take into account the fact that every five years 20% of the population of Montreal changes, while 43%

moves to a different neighbourhood. These activities primarily brought together actors from the health care network in addition to RIC members.

A discussion day, this time reserved solely for members of the RIC, permitted representatives of the Ministry of the Family (childcare services) and Ministry of Education to present their programs and overviews of the services they provided. However, the issues of childcare accessibility and quality and the development of kindergarten for four-year-olds were not specifically addressed in order to avoid undermining the spirit of dialogue, as partners were of different opinions as to the type of educational setting best suited to four-year-olds. The RIC also held another internal discussion on the day-to-day difficulties faced by community organizations.

These discussion days led to the creation of working groups, made up of RIC members and operating outside regular meetings, to explore certain topics in greater detail in preparation for the regional summit.

3.1.5. DPH Support for the Organization of Local Summits—2008–2009

Certain HSSCs perceived the mandate of organizing local summits as a command issued by the DPH while others, having been told of the survey in 2005, were ready and willing to mobilize their community. The HSSCs generally acknowledge that it was in their mandate to organize such a process in their community. However, they also recognized that the organization of the summit required leadership-sharing with the community and, with the exception of one territory, established organizing committees made up of intersectoral partners.

The DPH provided the 12 HSSCs with support, notably in the form of funding. At their request, it produced a guide for the organization of the events, suggesting strategic actors to invite and proposing a procedure to be followed and topics of discussion (Samson, 2008). To help actors assimilate the data, researchers put several tools at their disposal: (1) detailed reports by school board (5), school (203), HSSC and neighbourhood (12), a regional report, and a summary report; (2) a map of public early childhood programs in local territories; and (3) a summary table of school readiness and socioeconomic indices by HSSC territories and neighbourhoods.

In preparation for the local summits, the researchers made themselves available for two pre-summit meetings in each territory to discuss the survey data. These meetings permitted the researchers to learn of some criticisms of the survey, provoked notably by the somewhat alarmist coverage it had received in certain newspapers, and to prepare a response. They also provided an opportunity to discuss some of the surprising results in territories considered to be advantaged where the proportion of vulnerable children was high. During these discussions, a number of organizing committees asked the researchers to provide additional analyses for their HSSC, for children from immigrant backgrounds for example, or to map the schools that had or had not participated in the survey to provide them with a better understanding of unexpected results.

3.1.6. The Local Summits—2008–2009

The 12 local summits were held over a period of 10 months, and brought together approximately 100 people each. The events took various forms depending on the territory. The researchers presented the survey data as well as the issues they had identified. Some territories invited additional speakers while others presented complementary information such as the territory's socio-demographic profile and resources, or held forums with parents on preparing children for school. All offered a form of collective reflexivity through discussion workshops. There was greater mobilization in certain territories either due to their possessing more highly-developed collaborative practices, or because school readiness had been a local concern for several years, or because the results of the survey were so striking they gave rise to a sense of urgency. However, local summits in all territories attracted a diverse range of actors, including parents. RIC actors also took part, several in more than one territory, thereby ensuring local-regional alignment.

It goes without saying that ownership of the results took different forms in each territory, but the picture presented generally corresponded to actors' observations: (1) the data presented by neighbourhood revealed previously unsuspected or little mentioned zones of poverty and school readiness vulnerability; (2) the data presented in terms of the numbers of vulnerable children rather than simple percentages brought to light new priority intervention areas; and (3) the data on available public resources showed that some territories were particularly underequipped given their needs. This was true for example of reduced-contribution childcare: in two out of three HSSC territories, the percentage of available spaces was under 50%. Furthermore, although the *Education Act* of 1997 stipulates that all children from underprivileged backgrounds must have the possibility of attending kindergarten beginning at age four, 12 of the 60 schools serving the most disadvantaged areas in Montreal did not offer kindergarten for four-year-olds despite being located in areas where the proportion of at-risk children was higher than the Montreal average.

The numerous concerns raised by the picture presented were coloured by the socio-demographic characteristics of the territory, its history of mobilization, the intersectoral representativeness of the actors involved, and the range of services provided to families. However, in several territories, the survey re-opened the old divisive debate between schools and daycares as to where four-year-olds belong[2]. It also shone a light on the lack of formal links between early childhood resources and schools and the impact of this situation on children's transition to school. Bill 7, not yet adopted into law at the time of the summits, also raised a host of fears in all the territories. Several actors denounced the social public–philanthropic partnership that would touch on areas of public policy. Others questioned the political will to target children living in poverty while still others feared their voices would not be heard and that new orientations would upset the dynamics of local consultation and the configuration of services. Finally, the results raised parental doubts about the measures to be taken and concerns about the risk of stigmatizing certain children. Some feared decision-makers were moving towards early schooling by making kindergarten mandatory as of age four.

3.1.7. Preparation and Holding of the Montreal Summit—Spring 2009

The Montreal Summit was a regional event that brought the process to an end after 10 months of on-going local mobilization. Aware that local actors would want to have a voice at the summit, the RIC made the rounds beforehand to receive approval for its proposed program, and asked each of the 12 HSSC to write out three possible avenues for improving services. However, the RIC's program also offered the additional regional benefit of exploring issues affecting all territories, inspired by the working groups generated by the theme days.

The Montreal Summit of May 2009 brought together a variety of actors, of which the most numerous were the HSSCs, followed by community organizations and schools. The advantage of a regional forum was reflected in the question put to participants, *i.e.*, what regional and provincial mechanisms should be used to ensure a better fit between the needs of Montreal families and available services given the challenges posed by the diversity and mobility of Montreal families as well as the difficulty of reaching so-called "isolated" families. For each aspect of the question, a video produced with parents was presented, followed by a panel comprised of parents and early childhood professionals.

Local actors had high expectations for the RIC at the regional summit. They had mobilized to hold the local summits and proposed possible solutions, and they expected organizers to produce a summary of local demands and make commitments in line with the demands. The regional summit proved unsatisfactory on this level. No such summary was produced and no investment was announced *in situ* in

---

[2] In Quebec, most children start school with full-time kindergarten at age five. Children from underprivileged backgrounds have the possibility of attending part-time kindergarten beginning at age four. Twenty percent of Quebec children attend part-time kindergarten.

response to their concerns. Local actors saw no sign of the RIC's promised regional advantage, and had an impression of *déjà-vu*.

The regional summit concluded with a joint declaration by the RIC members in which they made a commitment to continue their efforts in favour of child development. In the aftermath of the summits, local actors said they were relieved no new program had been announced for top-down implementation. Otherwise, they said, what good would all their efforts have been if the outcome had been decided ahead of time?

Finally, the DPH produced a summary of all the written submissions produced during the process at both local and regional levels [33]. The analysis linked issues and solutions related to school readiness. Its first priority was to stress the necessity of taking action on family living conditions and the need to respect the fact that some families would first want to obtain support to meet their basic needs. It supported the adoption of non-blaming approaches with parents geared towards the creation of opportunities for families to come together rather than screening. Finally, it strongly emphasized the urgency of establishing formal links between early childhood resources and schools. It deplored the fact that most teachers had little knowledge of the preschool trajectories of the children they welcome into kindergarten. Parents are under a great deal of social pressure to ensure their children are "ready" when they start school, without really knowing what that means. The analysis served to guide the RIC in the development of its action plan.

3.2. The Post-Summit Collective Decision-Making Process: Developing a Solution Based on Early Childhood Services in the Community

The events that laid the foundation for the collective decision-making process regarding the development of solutions occurred simultaneously at regional and local levels following the regional summit of May 2009. The events involving the actor network will be examined first, followed by those concerned with solution implementation.

3.2.1. Regional and Local Actor Networks in the Post-Summit Period

In the two years following the regional summit, the 14 members of the RIC focused on giving the committee a clear identity, defining its mandate, and developing a strategic plan. They set up a coordination committee to ensure shared leadership among members and combat fears that had been present since the beginning of the process that the DPH would exercise too much influence over decisions. The RIC made changes to its composition to consolidate its partnership with other regional collaborative bodies, especially ones focusing on student retention and academic success. However, it was also faced with the withdrawal of one community actor that cited the actor's position against social public-private partnerships and its uneasiness with the fact that one of the RIC's main financial contributors was the product of such a partnership.

The post-summit period was marked by flagging collaboration between local and regional levels, as a result of regional actors' lack of support for local communities. Due to the importance of taking local concerns into account in establishing its guidelines, the RIC polled the 300 regional summit participants in the spring of 2010 regarding the primary courses of strategic action it should adopt. Following this sounding-out process, in June 2011 the RIC unveiled its strategic plan for 2010–2015 permitting regional actors to reconnect with local counterparts. In 2011 and 2012, the RIC conducted two projects to encourage renewed contact. The *Constellation* project was aimed at pooling and sharing experience and knowledge regarding difficult-to-reach families, while the objective of the *Basic Services Basket* project was to identify what parents and both local and regional actors would like to receive in terms of resources and basic services throughout the entire Montreal area. It addressed the problem of the unequal distribution of services among Montreal territories mentioned at the summits, as well as the issue of family mobility.

However, local actors' expectations of the regional level were high and remained unmet. On the one hand, they wanted the RIC to exercise political influence in situations where local entities were powerless. For example, they expected the RIC to appeal to public decision-makers to curb the proliferation of non-government-subsidized private daycares due to the absence of regulations governing such daycares and the lack of training of the educators who worked in them. Local actors also expected their regional counterparts in the RIC to promote actions designed to improve family living conditions. However, the position adopted by the RIC with regard to exercising political influence ensured it would never place its members in a difficult position, as they also had to answer to ministries responsible for public policies and programs. The regional actors concluded that they did not have the means to initiate action on these questions and agreed instead to join in lobbying efforts by other bodies. On the other hand, local actors requested that the regional level strive to ensure greater harmonization of early childhood funding. Such an expectation would undoubtedly be difficult to meet because any solution would signify a loss of autonomy for donors in terms of program definition and accountability. The arrival on the scene of actors issuing from public-philanthropic partnerships, with still more accounting mechanisms, did nothing to simplify the situation.

After the 2009 summits, local actors initially continued their work in the local committees set-up to organize the summits. After approximately a year, discussions were held in all territories, marking the dissolution of these committees whose work was then taken up by other local collaborative bodies in which the actors continued to work towards the priorities adopted. At the end of data collection in 2011, traces of the *Summit Initiative* were visible in all HSSC local action plans which served as the basis for continuation of community mobilization on this issue. The summits' influence was also apparent in certain local action plans that had previously focused on 6- to 12-year-olds but now incorporated activities targeting children ages 0 to five years. This was true for school boards, boroughs, and philanthropic partners.

These commitments signify the extension of the early childhood actor network, notably through connections with school boards, ardently desired by actors for many years, formalizing schools' desire to become involved. Henceforth, school principals had the approval of their regional and provincial counterparts to engage fully in early childhood discussions. The municipality, which the RIC had invited to participate from the very beginning, improved its relations with the community by developing connections with organizations. Due to their new outreach mandate, libraries were able to take an active role in consultations and participate in numerous intersectoral projects.

3.2.2. Survey and Summit Initiative Outcomes for Service Organization

Decision-making is primarily sectoral at government and regional levels. Actors identified a number of advances in which the contributions made by the survey and the Summit Initiative were apparent. The Government of Quebec's creation of the Fund for Early Childhood Development as part of a public-philanthropic partnership is unquestionably an important outcome. It allows for local funding of joint action and support for regional and interregional bodies that conduct knowledge- and practice-sharing activities, such as the RIC's Constellation and Basic Services Basket projects. In 2009, the Education Ministry launched its strategies for student academic success, which included pre-school actions involving the early childhood network. It used survey results, among other things, to establish selection criteria for territories targeted by its early literacy program. Finally, in 2010, it joined its counterparts in the health and family sectors to coproduce a guide to provide support for children's transition to school. On a regional level, the health, childcare, municipal and philanthropic sectors introduced additional resources, using survey data to better target the territories in which they should be implemented.

The process was also seen to have significant local outcomes, reflecting the DPH's desire, as stated at the opening of the summits, to take its cue from what works locally and further refine its interventions. Joint planning by local collaborative bodies was the principal *modus operandi* for collective decision-making to guide and coordinate the actions of public, public-philanthropic, and community actors. As in the problematization phase, collective reflection activities played an important role in the decision-making process during planning. Less documentation is available on the implementation or continuation of new services due to the study's short duration. Some of the outcomes took the form of initiatives on child language, motor and social development. Others were more general in nature, such as the creation of additional daycare spaces, parent-child workshops, a drop-in daycare, support for new arrivals, access to a reduced rate for city-run activities, and the establishment of a family outreach centre or social paediatric services. Of these, transition-to-school and literacy activities will be examined more closely as they were implemented in all territories. The full range of outcomes can be found in two general audience publications produced for the actors [13,14].

Transition-to-school actions were the result of the redefinition of preschool (0 to 5 years) guidelines adopted by the Ministry of Education. These actions include the use of school-transition tools. The aim of these tools was to provide a descriptive portrait of the child's overall development to foster discussion between community or childcare organizations and schools. They were also designed to ensure intervention continuity between networks. The tool is completed by the child's educator in the spring and given to the parents who are responsible for transmitting it to the school. To meet the needs of children not in childcare, school boards and community organizations offer parent-child workshops and educational kindergarten-preparation day camps. The camps have undergone considerable growth since 2008. In addition to the participation of the school and childcare communities, the implementation of new activities involves actors from community, health and municipal organizations.

The newly implemented early literacy programs are the product of a Ministry of Education emergent literacy program and the clear commitment of libraries to off-site programming. Librarians are present in the field and lead activities in a variety of different contexts, such as city parks and social housing complexes. Now books can be borrowed not only at libraries; but in community organizations, daycares, and parks as well, not to mention in the street through bookmobiles. The activities financed by the Ministry's early literacy program focus on integrating reading into children's and family activities. An example of such an activity might be setting up a reading corner in a HSSC waiting room. Books are also presented as gifts at immunization sessions and perinatal home visits.

The post-summit collective decision making process was devoted to developing local solutions specifically adapted to community needs. In a characteristic chain of events, the consolidation of the regional and local action networks, the provision of additional resources by government and regional sectoral decision-makers, and the ability of these networks to carry out on-going planning of the priorities established during the summit phase, would appear to have provided as the combined ingredients for the collective decisions.

4. Discussion

The initial focus of our study was to understand how a social health survey report can impel actors to mobilize to improve early childhood resources and services in communities. By using the actor-network theory, we wanted to establish how the problem under study—school readiness—was problematized in regional and local networks. We wanted to understand what encouraged mobilization, the processes by which the actor network expanded and was consolidated, the use it made of survey data, and the type of answers actors were able to supply. The study also enabled us to document precisely the issues raised by the EDI and the actions that ensued in the field of early childhood.

4.1. The Expansion and Consolidation of the Actor Network

Several of the quality attributes associated with collective action and decision-making processes were observed in the initiative under study here [34–36]. Such a broad mobilization process must be able to count on a system of action able to support it [37]. In this instance, Montreal's public health system, with its regional administration and 12 HSSCs provided this structure. Mobilization occurred within a dense, multi-sectoral network with a history of collaborative practices in the field of early education. We know that if a network is to be productive, it requires genuine, credible leadership [38]. Other actors in the network acknowledged that Montreal's public health system provided this leadership. If a collective decision-making process is to bring about change in a system of action, new knowledge and resources must be mobilized [35]. In this regard, in addition to survey data for small neighbourhood areas being made available in non-technical language, the DPH also provided logistical and financial support so HSSCs could organize local summits to foster ownership of and collective reflection on the results. To stimulate reflection and steer it towards public policies, the DPH took it upon itself to examine the survey results in light of the issues it had presented to the communities. It extended a more formal invitation to RIC members to present their opinions on these issues, thus ensuring they would be included on the Montreal summit agenda at the end of the data ownership process. Thus, the Montreal initiative succeeded in building the issue of school readiness into an important social issue by combining evidence with a knowledge-sharing process designed for a diverse target audience, which constituted the optimal conditions for making early childhood part of the political agenda [39]. Problematized in this manner, the issue of children's school readiness entreated new actors to engage in and endorse new roles in the search for solutions. The notion of translation in ANT appropriately reflects the process observed.

Even though a culture of intersectoral collaboration in early childhood was already present in three-quarters of Canadian municipalities well before the beginning of data collection using the EDI, the contribution of the results obtained and the accompanying mobilization acted as a catalyst for intersectoral action [23]. Montreal was no exception. While the *Summit Initiative* was part of consultation dynamic already well-established in municipalities, the consultation was transformed by the survey. First, because the survey results made it possible to quantify the situation, they gave child development a visibility and importance that was more compelling than before. This had an impact on early childhood actors who felt empowered to call attention to the situation of children under the age of five and their parents in other collaborative bodies to which they belonged concerned with social development, immigration, or school dropout for example. Next, in all territories the formation of intersectoral committees for local summit organization and follow-up resulted in the extension and consolidation of networks of partners. Finally, as a result of the actors having made actions targeting the transition from daycare to school a priority in the post-summit period, the two communities were brought closer together. All of these local collaborative transformations were fostered by the implementation of a regional intersectoral collaborative body at the time of the publication of the survey results, indicating a genuine commitment on the part of regional sectoral actors to claiming ownership of the results and following up with concrete action. For example, if boroughs and schools were as involved at the local level, it was because decision-makers in these sectors had made decisions accompanied by adequate funding to enable them to be agents of change. Thus, as observed by Janus [23], the results of Canada-wide surveys provided the raw material for creating dialogue and shifting decision-makers' focus to early childhood intervention. This was even truer of schools [40], as was observed in Montreal.

4.2. Survey Results as Planning Tools

Janus [23] observed that in many Canadian municipalities the activities established following the surveys were implemented in small territories, such as neighbourhoods, boroughs, or school districts. The same tendency was observed in Montreal, which is not surprising as actors were provided with a map of results by neighbourhood, HSSC territory, school board, and school. In addition to the practical knowledge they already possessed, the actors had everything, including socio-economic indicators and a map of public services, necessary to improve actions in priority areas. These areas were designated as such in part because of the survey results, but also because they were in outlying areas, lacked services, and had a high proportion of low-income and/or recently immigrated families. The outcome was new projects and services as well as the continuation of pre-existing programs, which, in light of the discussion initiated by the summits, were shown to be more than pertinent. Prior to the 2006 survey, intersectoral decision-makers undoubtedly had other sources of data at their disposal on which to base their decisions, from the Ministry of Education or of the Family for example, but the population data produced by the DPH served to as a bridge between different sources by shedding new light on the entire Montreal population of five-year-olds by territory. Thus, as in other Canadian provinces, the survey results were combined with other information for use as key criteria for the allocation of early childhood resources and of spaces in reduced-contribution childcare.

4.3. Outcomes for Action

It is more difficult to make a comparison with other Canadian municipalities with regard to outcomes for action as these are dependent on pre-existing services and, more broadly, on the public policies in place in the different provinces. Quebec's family policies stand apart in many ways from those in the rest of Canada, especially the universal daycare policy which has no equivalent in the other provinces, as well as the child assistance benefit and paid parental leave which are much more generous than elsewhere [41]. Nonetheless, of the outcomes inventoried on a Canada-wide basis by Janus [23], the most frequent were those associated literacy and designed to support cognitive and language development. A predominance of this type of projects was also observed in Montreal, as demonstrated by the early literacy activities. Just as important, transition-to-school activities also experienced a considerable boom, echoing the efforts made in several other Canadian municipalities to bridge the gap between the early childhood network and schools.

5. Conclusions

The preschool life of Quebec children is neither unique nor comprised of a single trajectory: some attend daycare, others start kindergarten at the age of four, and others remain at home until school starts for everyone at the age of five. In such a context, relying on intersectoral action ensures the provision of a greater range of services touching the various spheres of child development, better visibility in the community, and increased accessibility.

The results of this study show that considerable effort is being made locally to develop a range of services adapted to families' needs. Nonetheless, they raise important issues around public planning and call into question the ability of local communities to organize to meet the multiple needs of families and children. Central to the challenges they face is promoting equity in child development by striking a balance between local services and guaranteed access for families to equivalent services in all territories. This is in line with the recommendations made by Hertzman who, supported by a decade of EDI-based research, is ardently campaigning for universal access to early childhood services [42].

Acknowledgments: This study was made possible by a grant from the Canadian Institutes of Health Research (CIHR), 2009–2012—Population Health Intervention Research Initiative.

Author Contributions: Angèle Bilodeau and Isabelle Laurin, as co-principal investigators, contributed to the design of the study, the interpretation of the results and were principally involved with writing up the manuscript. Nadia Giguère was involved carrying out fieldwork and analysis. Louise Potvin contributed to the design of the study and the preparation of the manuscript.

Conflicts of Interest: The authors declare no conflict of interest.

Abbreviations

EDI   Early Development instrument;
DPH   Department of public health of the Montreal Health and Social Services Agency;
HSSC   Health and Social Services Centers;
RIC   regional intersectoral collaborative body.

References

1. Ron Haskins, Irwin Garfinkel, and Sara McLanahan. "Introduction: Two-generation mechanisms of child development." *Helping Parents Helping Children: Two-Generation Mechanisms: The Future of Children* 24 (2014): 3–13.
2. Nina Howe, and Larry Prochner. "Introduction." In *Recent Perspectives on Early Childhood Education and Care in Canada*. Edited by Nina Howe and Larry Prochner. Toronto: University of Toronto Press, 2014, pp. 1–11.
3. Margaret Norrie McCain, John Fraser Mustard, and Kerry McCuaig. *Le Point sur la Petite Enfance 3: Prendre des Decisions, Agir (Early Years Study 3: Making Decisions, Taking Action)*. Toronto: Margaret and Wallace McCain Family Foundation, 2011.
4. Miles Corak. "Income Inequality, Equality of Opportunity, and Intergenerational Mobility." *Journal of Economic Perspectives* 27 (2013): 79–102.
5. Aadrie Kusserow. *American Individualisms: Child Rearing and Social Class in Three Neighborhoods*. New York: Palmgrave Macmillan, 2004.
6. Sarah Theule Lubiensky. "Celebrating Diversity and Denying Disparaties: A Critical Assessment." *Educational Researcher* 32 (2003): 30–38.
7. Bruce Bradbury, Miles Corak, Jane Waldfogel, and Elizabeth Washbrook. "Inequality in Early Childhood Outcomes." In *From Parents to Children: The Intergenerational Transmission of Advantage.*. Edited by John Ermisch, Markus Jäntti, Jane Waldfogel and Liz Washbrook. New York: Russell Sage Foundation, 2012, pp. 87–119.
8. Neeraj Kaushal. "Intergenerational Payoffs of Education." *Helping Parents Helping Children: Two-Generation Mechanisms—The Future of Children* 24 (2014): 61–78.
9. Valerie E. Lee, and David Burkam. *Inequalities at the Starting Gate: Social Background Differences in Achievement as Children Begin School*. Washington: Economic Policy Institute, 2002.
10. Annie McEwen, and Jennifer Stewart. "The Relationship between income and children's outcomes: A synthesis of Canadian evidence." *Canadian Public Policy* 40 (2014): 99–109.

11. Magdalena Janus, and Dan R. Offord. "Development and Psychometric Properties of the Early Development Instrument (EDI): A Measure of Children's School Readiness." *Canadian Journal of Behavioural Science* 39 (2007): 1–22.
12. Magdalena Janus, Sally Brinkman, Erid Duku, Clyde Hertzman, Robert Santos, Joanne Schroeder, Mary Sayer, and Cindy Walsh. *The Early Development Instrument: A Population-based Measure for Communities—A Handbook on Development, Properties, and Use*. Hamilton: MacMaster University, 2007.
13. Isabelle Laurin, Angèle Bilodeau, Nadia Giguère, and Anouk Lebel. *Montreal Summits on School Readiness: Impacts on Mobilization. Focus on … Intersectoral Action*. Number 1. Montréal: Centre de Recherche Léa-Roback sur les Inégalités Sociales de Santé, 2014.
14. Isabelle Laurin, Angèle Bilodeau, Nadia Giguère, and Anouk Lebel. "Montreal Summits on School Readiness: Impacts on Service Organization." In *Focus on … Intersectoral Action*. Number 2. Montréal: Centre de Recherche Léa-Roback sur les Inégalités Sociales de Santé, 2014.
15. Isabelle Laurin, Sylvie Lavoie, Danielle Guay, Laurence Boucheron, Danielle Durand, and Nathalie Goulet. "Enquête sur le Développement des Enfants Montréalais à leur Entrée à l'école (Survey of the school readiness of Montreal children)." *Santé Publique* 24 (2012): 7–21.
16. Ministère de la Santéet des Services Sociaux. "Programme National de Santé Publique 2003–2012. Mise à Jour 2008 (Quebec Public Health Program, 2003–2012: Update for 2008)." Available online: http://www.quebecenforme.org/media/1387/programme_national_de_sante__publique_2003-2012.pdf (accessed on 4 December 2015).
17. Wilfried Kreisel, and Yasmin von Schirnding. "Intersectoral action for health: A cornerstone for health for all in the 21st Century." *World Health Statistics Quarterly* 51 (1998): 75–78.
18. Isabelle Laurin, Angèle Bilodeau, and Sébastien Chartrand. "Maturité scolaire et mobilisation communautaire: Étude rétrospective dans un quartier montréalais (School readiness and community mobilization: A retrospective study of a Montreal neighborhood)." *Canadian Journal of Public Health* 103 (2012): S32–38.
19. Louise Potvin, Sylvie Gendron, Angèle Bilodeau, and Patrick Chabot. "Integrating social theory into public health practice." *American Journal of Public Health* 95 (2005): 591–95.
20. Franklin Kutuadu, and Lori Baugh Littlejohns. *The School Readiness of Red Deer's Kindergarten Children: A Preliminary Report on the Results of the Early Development Instrument (EDI)*. Red Deer: Early Development Instrument (EDI), 2009.
21. Michael Quenell, and Kathryn Smart. *Understanding the Early Years Regina Community Mapping Report*. Regina: UEY Regina, 2010.
22. Mothercraft. "Early Development Instrument (EDI) 2010/11 Toronto Results (2011)." Available online: http://www.mothercraft.ca/assets/site/docs/resource-library/EDI/reports/201011_TorontoEDIReport.pdf (accessed on 4 December 2015).
23. Magdalena Janus. *Early Development Instrument: "From Results to Action Survey" Report*. Hamilton: Offord Centre for Child Studies, McMaster University, 2013.

24. Louise Potvin, and Sherry Bisset. "There Is More to Methodology than Method." In *Health Promotion Evaluation Practices in the Americas: Values and Research*. Edited by Louise Potvin and David V. McQueen. New York: Springer, 2008.
25. Michel Callon. "Éléments pour une sociologie de la traduction (Some Elements of a Sociology of Translation)." *L'année Sociologique* 36 (1986): 169–208.
26. Michel Callon. "Introduction." In *La Science et ses Réseaux. Genèse et Circulation des Faits Scientifiques*. Edited by Éditions La Découverte and Michel Callon. Paris: Éditions La Découverte, 1988, pp. 7–33.
27. Bruno Latour. *Changer de Société, Refaire de la Sociologie (Changing Societies, Rethinking Sociology)*. Paris: Éditions La Découverte, 2006.
28. Madeleine Akrich, Michel Callon, and Bruno Latour. "Sociologie de la traduction." In *Textes Fondateurs*. Paris: École des Mines de Paris, 2006.
29. Pierre Pluye, Louise Potvin, and Jean-Louis Denis. "La pérennisation organisationnelle des projets pilotes en promotion de la santé (The organizational perpetuation of health promotion pilot projects)." *Ruptures Revue Transdisciplinaire en Santé* 7 (2000): 99–113.
30. William Dab. "Réflexions sur les défis de la programmation en santé (Thoughts on the Challenges of Health Programming)." *Promotion et Éducation* 36 (2005): 169–208.
31. Louise Potvin, Angèle Bilodeau, and Sylvie Gendron. "Trois conceptions de la nature des programmes: Implication pour l'évaluation de programmes complexes en santé publique (Three perspectives on the nature of programs: Implications for the assessment of complex public health programs)." *The Canadian Journal of Program Evaluation* 26 (2012): 91–104.
32. Robert K. Yin. *Case Study Research*. Thousand Oaks: Sage, 1994.
33. Isabelle Laurin, Isabelle Samson, Sylvie Lavoie, Danielle Durand, and Laurence Boucheron. *Les Sommets sur la Maturité Scolaire—Document Synthèse de la Démarche Effectuée en 2008–2009 (The Summits on School Readiness: Summary Report on the 2008–2009 Process)*. Montreal: Direction de Santé Publique—Agence de la Santé et des Services Sociaux de Montréal, 2010.
34. Agence de Santé Publique du Canada. *Au Croisement des Secteurs—Expériences en Action Intersectorielle, en Politique Publique et en Santé (Crossing Sectors—Experiences in Intersectoral Action, Public Policy and Health)*. Ottawa: Agence de Santé Publique du Canada, 2007.
35. Angèle Bilodeau, Marilène Galarneau, Michel Fournier, and Louise Potvin. "L'Outil diagnostique de l'action en partenariat: Fondements, élaboration et validation (Diagnostic Tool for Partnership Action)." *Canadian Journal of public Health* 102 (2011): 298–302.
36. Roz D. Lasker, Elisa S. Weiss, and Rebecca Miller. "Partnership synergy: A practical framework for studying and strengthening the collaborative advantage." *Millbank Quarterly* 79 (2001): 179–205.
37. John M. Bryson, Barbara C. Crosby, and Melissa Middleton Stone. "The Design and implementation of Cross-Sector Collaborations: Propositions from the Literature." *Public Administration Review* 66 (2006): 44–55.

38. Henri Amblard, Philippe Bernoux, Gilles Herreros, and Yves François Livan. *Les Nouvelles Approches Sociologiques des Organisations*. Paris: Éditions du Seuil, 1996.
39. Aletha C. Huston. "From research to policy and back." *Child Development* 79 (2008): 1–12.
40. Janet Mort. *The Early Development Instrument (EDI) in British Columbia: Documenting Impact and Action in Schools, Communities and Childhood Development*. Vancouver: Council for Early Child Development, 2009.
41. Jane Jenson. "Early childhood learning and care: The route to meeting the major challenges." *Policy Options* 27 (2006): 55–58.
42. Clyde Hertzman. "Peut-on parler «d'équité dès le départ» au Canada (Is there equity from the start in Canada)? " *ISPP Pop Nouvelle* 22 (2010): 6–8.

Who Benefits from Public Healthcare Subsidies in Egypt?

Ahmed Shoukry Rashad and Mesbah Fathy Sharaf

Abstract: Direct subsidization of healthcare services has been widely used in many countries to improve health outcomes. It is commonly believed that the poor are the main beneficiaries from these subsidies. We test this hypothesis in Egypt by empirically analyzing the distribution of public healthcare subsidies using data from Egypt Demographic and Health Survey and Egypt National Health Accounts. To determine the distribution of public health care subsidies, we conducted a Benefit Incidence Analysis. As a robustness check, both concentration and Kakwani indices for outpatient, inpatient, and total healthcare were also calculated. Results show some degree of inequality in the benefits from public healthcare services, which varied by the type of healthcare provided. In particular, subsidies associated with University hospitals are pro-rich and have inequality increasing effect, while subsidies associated with outpatient and inpatient care provided by the Ministry of Health and Population have not been pro-poor but have inequality reducing effect (weakly progressive). Results were robust to the different analytical methods. While it is widely perceived that the poor benefit the most from health subsidies, the findings of this study refute this hypothesis in the case of Egypt. Poverty reduction measures and healthcare reforms in Egypt should not only focus on expanding the coverage of healthcare benefits, but also on improving the equity of its distribution.

Reprinted from *Soc. Sci.* Cite as: Rashad, A.S.; Sharaf, M.F. Who Benefits from Public Healthcare Subsidies in Egypt? *Soc. Sci.* **2015**, *4*, 1162–1176.

---

1. Introduction

The World Health Organization (WHO) has been calling for a sustainable and equitable financing and delivery of healthcare services. This is to improve access to healthcare, offer greater financial protection to the poor and to combat poverty, hunger, and diseases, which are key ingredients of the United Nations Millennium Development Goals [1].

Adequate access to healthcare services is crucial for increasing productivity of the labor force, and hence economic growth. In the absence of universal health insurance coverage, subsidization of healthcare becomes essential to ensure that the poor can afford access to health services. Direct subsidization of healthcare services has been widely used as an effective policy instrument to improve health levels in many developing countries. Health subsidies could reduce income inequalities if the subsidy is benefiting the poor more than rich. Thus, the effect of the subsidies on income distribution depends on the distribution of the subsidization benefits across different economic classes.

Egypt has been adopting a subsidized healthcare system for several decades. It is commonly believed that the poor are the main beneficiaries from these subsidies. The objective of the current study is to test this hypothesis in Egypt by empirically analyzing the distribution of public healthcare subsidies using nationally representative data from Egypt Demographic and Health Survey.

Following the establishment of the Republic of Egypt in 1952, the new socialist regime has relied on a redistribution system that promoted a minimum standard of living by providing universal subsidies of basic consumption goods [2]. Egypt has one of the biggest subsidy programs that cover food and energy on a massive scale. In the health sector, the government of Egypt has pledged to provide free healthcare to all citizens. Right of access to healthcare is a constitutional right in Egypt, and the government uses general tax revenue to provide subsidized healthcare services.

Over the period 2000 to 2009, public health spending in Egypt accounted for 6% of the total public spending. This is far behind the Abuja target of allocating 15% of total government spending to health. The subsidized health system is under continuous population pressure resulting from the significant increase in life expectancy and the high fertility rates. Consequently, this has led to increasing use of private health facilities, which require fees [3,4]. To obtain adequate healthcare, many households in Egypt rely on out-of-pocket financing which increases the risk of becoming impoverished if the out-of-pocket payments were substantial and for prolonged periods. Excessive reliance on out-of-pocket payments may increase inequalities in access to healthcare and could also increase intergenerational inequality if the households' ability to invest in their children's health and education is reduced [5,6]. Statistics show that out-of-pocket payments are the principle mean of financing healthcare in Egypt. According to the National Health Accounts, in 2008, out-of-pocket payments accounted for 60% of health spending. The seventh round of the Egyptian Family Observatory Survey revealed that 80% of households have at least one member covered by public health insurance. However, the survey pointed out that only 25% of the insured households are benefiting from it due to low quality services and excessive red tape. This suggests that health shocks may push non-poor into poverty and exacerbate the poverty of the poor [7].

To the best of our knowledge, this study is among the first to assess the distribution of government health sector subsidies across economic classes in Egypt. To evaluate whether public health spending is pro-poor or pro-rich, the study uses Benefit Incidence Analysis (BIA) [8–10]. BIA is a commonly used accounting procedure that helps determine who gets how much of the amount the government spends providing healthcare to the population.

The paper is organized as follows: Section 2 presents a brief review of the related literature. Section 3 provides an overview on the structure of the healthcare system in Egypt. The data is described in Section 4, and the empirical methodology is presented in Section 5. Empirical results are discussed in Section 6. Section 7 summarizes the findings of the paper and discusses some policy recommendations. Section 8 concludes the paper.

2. Literature Review

Health shocks could increase households' vulnerability and disrupt their livelihood. To make healthcare services affordable, many countries adopt a subsidized universal healthcare system with the pre-assumption that the poor are the ones who benefit the most. The importance of an equitable distribution of the benefits from public healthcare subsidies stems from the fact that with no adequate access of healthcare services, vulnerable households may resort to out-of-pocket payments which increases the risk of becoming impoverished if the payments were substantial and for prolonged periods[1]. In a cross country study of 11 Asian countries, Van Doorslaer *et al.* [11] examined whether out-of-pocket healthcare payments exacerbate poverty. They found that poverty estimates after accounting for the out-of-pocket healthcare payments were much higher than the conventional estimates, ranging from an additional 1.2% of the population in Vietnam to 3.8% in Bangladesh. In a recent study, Rashad and Sharaf [12] found empirical evidence that out-of-pocket health expenditures pushed 6% of the Egyptian households to encounter financial catastrophe, and 7.4% of the households fell below the poverty line after controlling for healthcare expenditures. They also found that rural households are more likely to incur catastrophic health expenditure when compared to urban households.

Several studies have examined the distribution of benefits from public healthcare subsidies in a wide range of countries with mixed findings[2]. For example, in a cross-country study, O'Donnell *et al.* [8] reported substantial variation, across 11 Asian countries, in the incidence of public healthcare subsidies. The study revealed that public health subsidy is strongly pro-poor in Hong Kong, moderately pro-poor in Malaysia and Thailand, evenly distributed in Sri Lanka, while it is mildly pro-rich in Vietnam. In the remainder of the low-income countries and provinces examined, the better-off receive substantially more of the subsidy than do the poor. In another cross-country study of 69 countries, Wagstaff *et al.* [14] estimated the pro-poorness

---

[1] For a recent review of literature on the economic impacts of health shocks on households in low and middle income countries see Alam and Mahal [6].

[2] For a recent systematic review of the literature on the equity aspects in the distribution of public health sector expenditure in low- and middle-income countries see Anselmi *et al.* [13].

average, government health expenditures are pro-rich. At the country level, in the majority of countries, government health expenditure is neither pro-rich nor pro-poor, while in a small minority it is pro-rich, and in an even smaller minority it is pro-poor. In addition, government health spending on contracted private facilities are pro-rich for all types of care, and in almost all Asian countries government health spending overall is significantly pro-rich. Moreover, they found that at the country level, the pro-poorness of government health spending is positively correlated with per-capita GDP, per-capita government health spending, and with six measures of the quality of a country's governance, while negatively correlated with the share of government facility revenues coming from user fees.

In addition to cross country studies, a growing number of country-specific studies have examined the distribution and equity aspects of public healthcare subsidies in a wide range of countries, during different periods, and using different estimation techniques with similarly mixed findings (e.g., [6,15–18]). For instance, Akazili *et al.* [15] conducted an assessment of the financing and benefit incidence of health services in Ghana and found that the healthcare financing system is progressive, while the distribution of total benefits from both public and private health services is pro-rich. However, public sector district-level hospital inpatient care is pro-poor and benefits of primary-level healthcare services are relatively evenly distributed. The study also reported a number of access constraints which contribute to inequities in the distribution of health service benefits in Ghana.

In another study, Limwattananon *et al.* [17] found that public subsidies to healthcare, both outpatient (OP) and inpatient (IP) services to public hospitals and health facilities, in Thailand was pro-poor between 2003 and 2009, which preferentially benefited the poorer quintiles. Burger *et al.* [16] investigated whether public health spending and access to healthcare services in South Africa have become more or less pro-poor over time. They found that public health spending became more pro-poor between 1993 and 2008, with an increase in the share of public clinic and hospital spending going to the poor. In addition, there were improvements in both financial and physical access to public health services which significantly helped poor households who are more frequent users of public hospitals and clinics than those who are more affluent. Onwujekwe *et al.* [9] found evidence that although coverage of priority public health services were well below target levels in Nigeria, the poorer quintiles and rural residents that are in greater need received more net benefits from provision of these health services.

Using BIA, Anselmi *et al.* [19] assessed horizontal and vertical equity in the geographic allocation of recurrent expenditure for outpatient healthcare across districts in Mozambique between 2008 and 2011. They found a pro-rich distribution of government spending, driven by pro-rich service utilization. Though an improvement towards horizontal and vertical equity, in both government and donor expenditure, took place between 2008 and 2011, inequities in the distribution of expenditure across beneficiaries persisted and were driven by inequities in service use.

In a recent study, Chen *et al.* [18] examined how the benefits from government healthcare subsidies in China are distributed. Using a BIA, they found an inequitable distribution of government healthcare subsidies during the period 2002 to 2007, where high-income individuals generally reap larger benefits from the subsidized healthcare system. Although greater healthcare subsidies were concentrated among the rich and did not demonstrate inequality-reducing effects in different regions over the studied years, some policy reforms along with the decrease in out-of pocket-payments and the rising allocation of government healthcare resources to healthcare facilities widened access and improved the opportunity to receive healthcare benefits all of which reduced inequity.

This paper contributes to the extant literature by providing empirical evidence on the distribution of public healthcare subsidies by focusing on the specific case of Egypt on which limited research has been conducted. To our knowledge, only one related study has investigated the distributional aspect of public health care expenditure in Egypt. In an earlier study, Rannan-Eliya *et al.* [20], combined data from the national health accounts, and micro data from the National Household Health Utilization and Expenditure Survey conducted in 1994, to examine the degree of inequality in the distribution of health expenditures in Egypt. The incidence of overall health expenditures in Egypt was found to be progressive. They concluded that the social insurance programs in Egypt, and the use of cost recovery in some public sector institutions contributed to greater inequality in the access to health care resources, both when evaluated by the level of income, and gender. The 1994–1995 expansion of social health insurance coverage to children has not improved the distribution of health care spending in favor of lower income households. The current study extends the earlier study of Rannan-Eliya *et al.* [20] by using an up to data from the Egyptian Demographic and Health Survey (EDHS), and using a BIA.

In the next section, we will shed the light on the structure of the healthcare system in Egypt.

3. Structure of the Healthcare System in Egypt

Egypt has a highly pluralistic healthcare system, with several different public and private providers and financing agents [3]. Public health providers include the Ministry of Health and Population (MOHP) and other organizations that receive budgetary support from the government general revenues. The MOHP operates a large network of health facilities that offer comprehensive healthcare to all Egyptians at highly subsidized rates. It owns more than 441 hospitals and 4839 primary healthcare centers. Eighty percent of MOHP's services are free and the rest requires some user fees. In addition to out of pocket payments and donations, the vast majority of MOHP funding comes from the Ministry of Finance. University hospitals are important health providers that provide primary, secondary, and tertiary treatment. They are autonomous facilities affiliated to individual universities and fall under the responsibility of the Ministry of Higher Education. The number of University Hospitals is 76 hospitals in 2008. Funding to University hospitals comes mainly from the Ministry of Finance through the Ministry of Higher Education and 30% comes from user fees. They are highly concentrated in Cairo and urban areas.

In addition to MOHP and University hospitals, Teaching Hospitals and Institutes Organization (THIO), Curative Care Organization (CCO) and the Health Insurance Organization are additional key healthcare providers. They are quasi-governmental organizations. Teaching Hospitals and Institutes Organization runs 11 general teaching hospitals and 20 research institutes which provides primary, secondary, and tertiary services. Half of the THIO's services are free of charge, and it serves a small proportion of the population due to its small size. It receives funding from the Ministry of Finance, MOHP and private firms through contracts, international donors through grants, the Health Insurance Organization through contracts and direct user fees. CCO is a non-profit organization under the authority of MOHP. It operates 11 urban hospitals that provide a comprehensive range of curative care services mainly to urban residents. It does not receive any subsidy from the Government, and hence it relies on 100% cost recovery. The Health Insurance Organization is an independent public organization under the authority of the MOHP. It provides compulsory insurance to formal sector workers, widows and pensioners, school children and newborns. It is funded mainly from insurance premiums and co-payments, and it covers 55% of the population. However, less than half of the insured are really benefiting from the insurance scheme [21].

Figure 1 depicts the percentage of delivery in a Health Facility by wealth quintiles in 2008. As evident from the figure, there are large disparities in healthcare utilization across wealth quintiles. For example, women in the richest quintile are more than twice as likely as women in the poorest quintile to deliver in a health facility. Based on a survey, 70 percent of poor households mentioned financial cost as a significant impediment to healthcare [2].

Despite subsidization, statistics show that the utilization of MOHP outpatient facilities is very low. The most striking fact about the choice of a healthcare provider is the high use of private healthcare among the poor. Figure 2 displays the choice of a provider for outpatient care by income quintiles. The private sector dominates the provision of outpatient care even among the poor. For households in the poorest quintile, 15% of all outpatient visits occurred in MOHP outpatient facilities, while 70% occurred in the private sector. The utilization of MOHP outpatient facilities steadily decreases with income. A similar pattern is observed for inpatient care

(Figure 3). The utilization of MOHP inpatient facilities is more frequent than MOHP outpatient facilities, which is likely due to the high fees associated with inpatient care at private facilities. Private sector is the preferred provider for inpatient care for the wealthiest quintile and even for the insured patients if they can afford it.

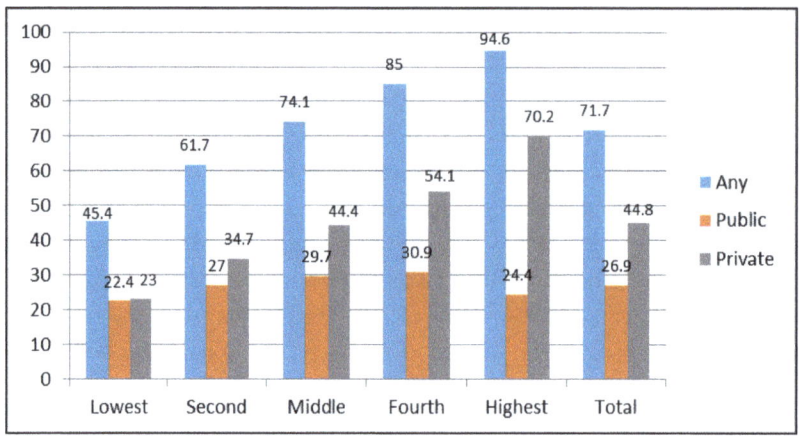

Figure 1. Delivery in a health facility by wealth quintiles in 2008. Source: Egypt Demographic and Health Survey [22].

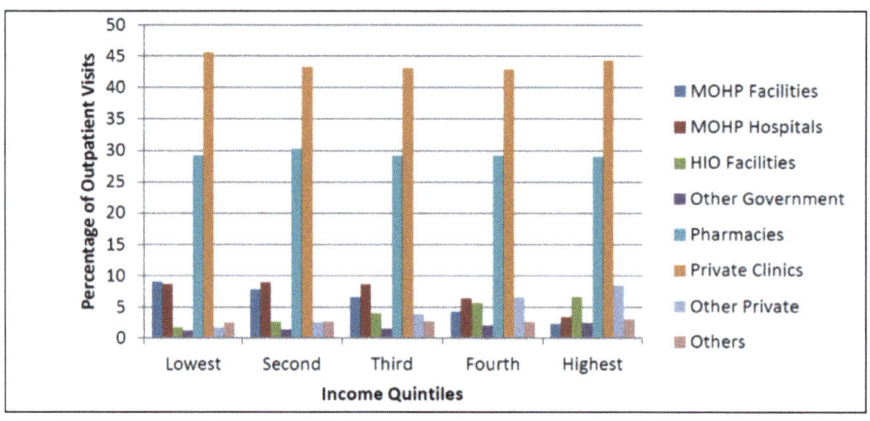

Figure 2. Choice of outpatient care provider by income quintile. Source: Egypt National Health Accounts [23].

It is difficult to run a BIA using data on quasi-governmental organizations, as they raise funds from several sources, and it is not possible to identify the subsidized patients from the non-subsidized ones. Consequently, in this study, BIA is limited to public health providers, both MOHP and University hospital, as both mainly get funding from the general tax revenue, and both constitute the biggest public health providers in Egypt in terms of coverage.

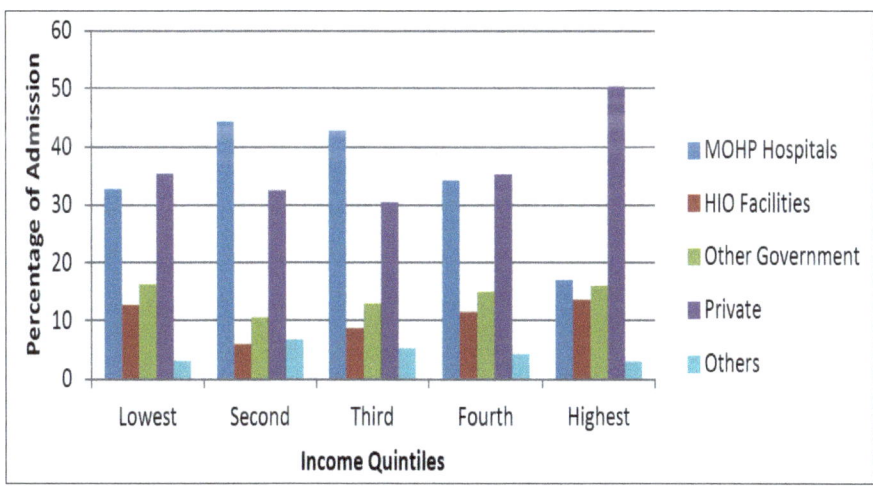

Figure 3. Inpatient care provider by income quintile. Source: Egypt National Health Accounts [23].

Private for-profit-health providers and other non-profit organizations that are not subsidized from the government revenue are not taken into account. Three categories of healthcare services are explored in the BIA: ambulatory visits to MOHP, hospital stays in MOHP, and hospital stays in University Hospitals.

4. Data

The main data set of this paper is the Egyptian Demographic and Health Survey (EDHS). The EDHS is a micro data survey implemented in 2008 and covers a nationally representative sample of 12,008 individuals. The survey collects a wide range of vital information on health related behavior, as well as corresponding economic and socio-demographic variables. Of particular importance, the EDHS includes information on outpatient visits to healthcare providers, hospital stays, and health expense incurred [22]. The survey distinguishes between public and private care and collects information on the level of household ownership, which is used to construct a measure of living standard based on the principal component analysis.

To conduct a BIA, we need the amount of public spending on each type of healthcare service for which utilization data are available on the survey. Data on public spending on healthcare are computed from the Egyptian National Health Accounts [23] (Table 1)[3].

Table 1. Public health spending, in Egyptian Pounds, for the year 2008.

Health Provider	Public Expenditure	Out of Pocket Payments	Unit Cost
MOHP Hospitals	3,819,458,728,00	288,049,928,00	281
University Hospitals	2,638,095,984,00	294,610,573,00	536
Outpatient care	2,180,591,664,00	527,439,388,00	60

Source: Egyptian National Health Accounts [23].

Conducting the BIA requires a health survey that has information on the utilization of the entire population of all types of healthcare, and all types of health facilities. In general, the standard Demographic and Health Survey (DHS) questionnaire cannot be used in conducting a BIA, as it does not gather enough information on health care utilization, or on the expenses incurred as it is too partial [24]. However, EDHS for the year 2008, has a special feature that makes it unique. It collects information on different types of health care utilization prior to the interview and on expenses households may have incurred for health services [22]. Consequently, the paper has greatly benefited from this exceptional round, and performed the BIA for Egypt using this special round. Given what has been stated, it would be obvious now why the current study has used the EDHS round for the year 2008, instead of using the most recent round of 2014.

5. Methodology: Benefit Incidence Analysis

To determine whether public healthcare spending in Egypt is pro-poor or pro-rich, we use the BIA[4]. The BIA is a commonly used accounting procedure, which helps determine the share of the different recipients in the healthcare expenditure provided by the government.

The first step of the BIA is estimation of the service-specific subsidy received by a patient which is calculated as in Equation (1).

$$s_{ki} = q_{ki} c_{kj} - f_{ki} \qquad (1)$$

---

[3] Unit cost is assumed to be the same for a given type of service. Additionally, due to data limitations, variations in the quality of health care services across regions are not captured in the analysis.
[4] For a more technical discussion of the BIA and its associated assumptions see Wagstaff [10].

where q_{ki} is the quantity of health service k utilized by patient i. f_{ki} is the fee paid for service k by patient i. c_{kj} is the cost per unit of health service k at region j. Unit cost is calculated by dividing total spending on service k by the weighted quantity of utilization provided in the survey as in Equation (2).

$$c_k = \frac{S_k + F_k}{\sum q_{ki}} \tag{2}$$

where S_k and F_k are the sum of government subsidies and out of pocket payments on service k respectively divided by the aggregate utilization $\sum q_{ki}$.

The total amount of the subsidy received by patient i is calculated as in Equation (3).

$$s_i = \sum_k \alpha_k \left(q_{ki} c_{kj} - f_{ki} \right) \tag{3}$$

α_k standardizes the recall period across different types of healthcare services. It is an equal one if the recall period is one year and equals 13 for a four-week recall period.

After estimating the total amount of the subsidy received by each individual in the sample, the next step is to examine the distribution of the subsidy across the different income quintiles. A concentration index is used to determine whether the subsidization of healthcare is pro-poor or pro-rich. The concentration index (CI) is a quantification of the degree of economic related inequality in the variable of interest. A positive CI indicates pro-rich distribution of subsidies, and a negative CI reflects pro-poor distribution. The higher the absolute value of the CI, the greater is the degree of concentration of subsidies among the economic group. CI of subsidies could get more pro-poor either due to low utilization of public health facilities by the rich or higher concentration of user fees among the rich. The CI is calculated as in Equation (4):

$$CI = \frac{2}{\mu} \, Cov \, (S, W) \tag{4}$$

In Equation (4), S is the amount of the subsidy received by individual i and μ is its mean, while W is a measure of living standard. The concentration index depends on the covariance between the amount of the subsidy received and its association with the measure of living standard. In addition to the CI, the concentration curve is used to illustrate the share of subsidies received by cumulative proportions of individuals in the population across the income distribution.

The CI and the concentration curve are powerful tools for assessing the distribution of health sector subsidies. However, visual inspection of concentration curve is not sufficient to conclude whether the subsidies are pro-poor or pro-rich. A formal test of statistical dominance is necessary to definitively conclude whether health sector subsidies benefit the poor more or not. According to the concentration curve dominance test, the concentration curve for outpatient care is statistically pro-poor if at least one quintile point at which the concentration curve for outpatient care lies significantly above the 45 degree line, and there is no quintile point at which the 45 degree line lies above the concentration curve [8].

In addition to the concentration curve dominance test, Kakwani's progressivity index is also used as a robustness check. This index evaluates whether the health sector subsidies reduce inequality (weak progressivity) by comparing income distribution to subsidies' distribution. It is equal to the difference between the subsidies concentration index and the Gini index, and it ranges between -2 and 1. Data for the Gini coefficient and income shares are obtained from the World Development Indicators issued by the World Bank. All analyses and estimations are population weighted using the sampling weights provided in the survey.

6. Results

Table 2 reports the average subsidy received by each wealth quintile for inpatient admission at University hospitals, outpatient visit to MOHP, and hospital stays at MOHP, respectively. The table also displays the share of each wealth quintile in the public subsidies in relative terms, as well as results of the different tests of dominance.

Results show that subsidies for University hospitals increase with wealth level. The fourth wealth quintile is benefiting six times higher than the poorest wealth quintile. On the contrary, public subsidies for ambulatory care in MOHP and inpatient care in MOHP hospitals are inversely related to wealth level.

Households at the poorest wealth quintile receive 40% of the public subsidies associated with ambulatory care, while households at the richest quintile receive 16% of these subsidies. A similar pattern is observed for inpatient care at MOHP hospitals. For University hospitals, the poorest quintile receives only 11% of the public subsidies, while the fourth quintile alone receives 67% of the subsidies.

Table 2 shows a positive CI for University hospitals, which suggests that subsidies associated with University hospitals are strongly concentrated among the rich. This result was further confirmed by the positive sign of the Kakwani index for inpatient admission at University hospitals. This indicates that subsidies associated with hospital care at University hospitals increased the income gap between the rich and the poor.

On the other hand, the concentration indices for outpatient visits and inpatient care at MOHP are both negative, indicating that the public subsidies for these healthcare services are pro-poor. Overall, health sector subsidies seem slightly pro-poor, as the CI of total subsidies is almost equal to zero. Results of the Kakwani indices for outpatient visits and inpatient care at MOHP are both negative, which are in line with the results of the CI. This indicates that subsidies associated with the MOHP, for outpatient and inpatient visits, reduce the income gap between the poor and the rich.

Table 2. Distribution of healthcare subsidies in Egyptian pounds.

	Income	University Hospitals	MOHP Outpatient	MOHP Inpatient	Total Subsidies
Mean subsidy					
Lowest quintile	5153	20.05	35.94	103.81	159.60
		(20.05)	(5.58)	(38.82)	(43.97)
Poorest 40%	7216	5.95	34.22	52.32	92.33
		(5.95)	(4.42)	(23.99)	(25.51)
Poorest 60%	9086	12.28	32.06	44.64	88.91
		(7.60)	(4.23)	(20.41)	(22.55)
Poorest 80%	11,687	121.09	22.14	16.61	159.75
		(69.35)	(3.57)	(12.38)	(70.50)
Highest quintile	22,341	19.77	24.23	42.09	86.01
		(19.77)	(4.81)	(20.54)	(28.98)
Total	11,192	35.82	29.72	51.87	117.30
		(15.10)	(2.04)	(11.09)	(18.87)
Shares (%)					
Lowest quintile	9.3	11.2	24.1	40	27.2
		(10.92)	(3.19)	(10.86)	(6.70)
Poorest 40%	13	3.3	23.0	20.2	15.8
		(3.50)	(2.73)	(8.36)	(4.41)
Poorest 60%	16.4	6.9	21.6	17.2	15.2
		(4.89)	(2.64)	(7.36)	(4.04)
Poorest 80%	21	67.6	14.9	6.4	27.2
		(16.84)	(2.28)	(4.66)	(9.23)
Highest quintile	40.3	11.0	16.3	16.2	14.7
		(10.81)	(2.90)	(7.39)	(4.79)
Total	100	100	100	100	100
Test of Dominance					
Against 45 degree line		None	None	None	None
Against Income distribution		None	D−	D+	D+
Concentration Index		0.3182	−0.1051	−0.2168	−0.0252
		(0.15)	(0.04)	(0.12)	(0.09)
Kakwani Index		0.1	−0.309	−0.51	−0.31

Note: Total refers to overall subsidies, standard errors are in parenthesis. None indicates that the concentration curve is indistinguishable from the 45 degree line or Lorenz curve. D− and D+ indicate that the concentration curve is significantly distinguishable from the compared distribution.

Results of the dominance tests, conducted to investigate whether health sector subsidies are significantly pro-poor at the 5% significance level, fail to reject the null hypothesis that the concentration curves are indistinguishable from the line of equality. This indicates that public healthcare subsidies are not pro-poor. However, testing the concentration curves against the income distribution shows that the concentration curves for outpatient and inpatient care at the MOHP dominate the income distribution curve. This suggests that subsidies associated with the MOHP are inequality-reducing (weakly progressive).

Figure 4 depicts the concentration curves for health sector subsidies and shows that the concentration curves for outpatient and inpatient care at MOHP are lying above the line of equality, which means that the poor benefit more from public subsidies than the rich. In contrast, the concentration curve for university hospitals lies below the line of equality, which indicates that the rich households benefit more from the public subsidies for university hospitals. The concentration curve for total public healthcare subsidies is slightly above the 45 degree line for the first two quintiles and, as we move farther, it is almost on the top of the 45 degree line.

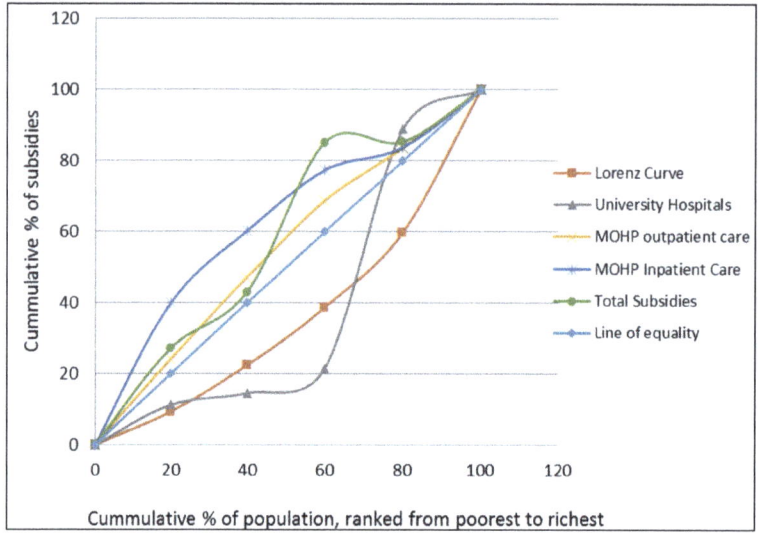

Figure 4. Concentration curves for health sector subsidies.

7. Discussion and Policy Implications

Egypt has been adopting a subsidized healthcare system for decades. This paper examined whether public healthcare subsidies in Egypt are pro-poor or pro-rich. Results show that public subsidies to healthcare services in Egypt are not pro-poor, meaning that subsidies tend to benefit wealthier groups more than the poorer groups. Under less restrictive assumption, in which the distribution of subsidies is compared to income distribution, the BIA showed that subsidies associated with the MOHP have inequality-reducing effect (weakly progressive). University hospitals' subsidies are mainly benefiting the rich and did not contribute to closing the income gap.

Previous studies have documented a number of access constraints which contribute to inequities in the distribution of health service benefits. These include long queues, long waiting hours, and inadequate staff and equipment in healthcare facilities especially in rural areas [15,25,26].

Geographical access is a major challenge, particularly for rural populations. This could explain why subsidies associated with University hospitals in Egypt are pro-rich. The poor are more likely to live in rural communities, while University hospitals are in urban areas. In addition, University hospitals require some sort of user fees and the poor are most affected by high user fees. This implies that user fees would reduce access to health-care more for the poor than for the better off. Therefore, the burden of user fees and transportation costs could be among the primary reasons for the inequitable distribution of the University hospitals' subsidies in Egypt. Red tape and long waiting lists for many healthcare services especially surgeries, medical exams and hospitalization have also been reported as major access barriers by the poor. The seventh round of the Egyptian Family Observatory Survey revealed that only 25% of households who are covered by public health insurance are benefiting from it due to low quality services and excessive red tape. Statistics from Egypt National Health Accounts show that in 2008, only 8.1% and 21% of the insured individuals use Health Insurance Organization (HIO) facilities for outpatient and inpatient healthcare. Insured individuals reported several reasons for not using HIO facilities: distance was cited by 18% of the individuals, 35 percent cited the long waiting time, and 44 percent cited lower-quality services [23].

To ensure an equitable distribution of health service benefits, poverty reduction policies should tackle the access constraints that affect the distribution of benefits. One policy measure for improving the distribution of subsidies is targeting health subsidies more toward illness associated with poverty. For instances, poor housing, poor nutrition, and lack of sanitation are associated with certain types of diseases. The government could link subsidies to these types of diseases. We recommend re-engineering the allocation of health sector subsidies toward healthcare services and facilities that are mostly used by the poor households. Another policy option is reducing the user fees associated with University hospitals, especially for the poor, and redirecting subsidies from University hospitals to MOHP facilities, which are the main source of healthcare services for the poor and rural residents.

Addressing the problems associated with the HIO facilities, and improving the quality of the provided services could also be an essential step to achieve an equitable distribution of public healthcare subsidies and increase the usage of HIO facilities. This has to be supplemented with improved focus on primary care and immunization, especially in rural and remote communities, in which the Non-Governmental Organizations (NGOs) and the private sector could play a vital role. In a review of the contracting experiences in 10 low-income countries, Loevinsohn and Harding [27] found that contracting with NGOs and the private sector to deliver healthcare or nutrition services was in general effective. Contractors, both NGOs and private healthcare providers, are more efficient than government agencies in terms of quality and coverage of the provided healthcare services and were more cost-effective. There is substantial empirical evidence that contracting increases accessibility, utilization level and coverage of healthcare services [28]. Levin and Kaddar [29] conducted a literature review on the role of the private sector in the provision of immunization services in low-and middle-income countries. They found that in low-income countries, the private for-profit sector is contributing to immunization service delivery and helping to extend access to traditional vaccines. In middle-income countries, the private for-profit sector facilitates early adopted new vaccines and technologies before introduction and generalization by the public sector. They also found that the not-for-profit sector plays an important role in extending access to traditional Expanded Program on Immunization (EPI) vaccines in low-income countries especially in rural and remote areas.

The current study has some limitations that warrant acknowledgment. First, the cross sectional nature of the used survey limits the ability to infer causality and to examine how the equity aspects of public subsidies evolve over time. The availability of longitudinal data in the future would stimulate further research to study the dynamics of the problem under investigation which will help design more effective policies to tackle it. Second, there could be other confounding factors that affect the benefit incidence of public health subsidies which we did not control for such as differences in geographical access to healthcare facilities, variations in the quality of healthcare services across communities, and patient satisfaction.

Poverty reduction measures and healthcare reforms in Egypt should not only focus on expanding the coverage but also on improving the equity of distribution of healthcare benefits.

8. Conclusions

We found robust evidence that in Egypt, public healthcare subsidies associated with University hospitals are pro-rich and have inequality increasing effect, while subsidies associated with outpatient and inpatient care provided by the MOHP have not been pro-poor but have inequality reducing effect (weakly progressive). While it is widely perceived that the poor benefit the most from the health subsidies, the findings of this study refute this hypothesis in the case of Egypt. Poverty reduction measures and healthcare reforms in Egypt should not only focus on expanding the coverage of healthcare benefits but also on improving the equity of its distribution. Addressing the problems associated with HIO facilities, improving the quality of the provided services, and contracting with NGOs and the private sector to deliver healthcare or nutrition services, especially in rural and remote areas, could also be a promising policy option.

Acknowledgments: The authors would like to thank the two anonymous referees and the academic editor of this journal for the invaluable comments and suggestions which have substantially improved the manuscript.

Author Contributions: Both Authors contributed equally to the conceptualization, design and composition of the paper. Both authors read and approved the final manuscript.

Conflicts of Interest: The authors declare no conflict of interest.

References

1. World Health Organization. "Sustainable Health Financing, Universal Coverage and Social Health Insurance—Resolution WHA583. 33." 2005. Available online: http://www.who.int/health_financing/documents/cov-wharesolution5833/en/ (accessed on 10 October 2014).
2. Matteo Morgandi, Joana Silva, and Victoria Levin. *Inclusion and Resilience: The Way Forward for Social Safety Nets in the Middle East and North Africa, Overview*. Washington: World Bank, 2012.
3. Fatma El-Zanaty, and Ann Way. "Egypt: DHS, 2005—Final Report." February 2006. Available online: http://dhsprogram.com/publications/publication-fr176-dhs-final-reports.cfm (accessed on 20 November 2014).
4. Lenka Benova, Oona M. R. Campbell, and George B. Ploubidis. "Socio-economic gradients in maternal and child health-seeking behaviours in Egypt: Systematic literature review and evidence synthesis." *PLoS ONE* 9 (2014): e93032.
5. Ke Xu, David B. Evans, Guido Carrin, Ana Mylena Aguilar-Rivera, Philip Musgrove, and Timothy Evans. "Protecting households from catastrophic health spending." *Health Affairs* 26 (2007): 972–83.
6. Khurshid Alam, and Ajay Mahal. "Economic impacts of health shocks on households in low and middle income countries: A review of the literature." *Global Health* 10 (2014): 21.
7. Information and Decision Support Center. "Bank of Surveys: Eighth Round of the Egyptian Family Observatory Survey." 2010. Available online: http://surveysbank.org.eg/Cod_Surveys/SurveyDetails_dtl.aspx?Survey_id=350URL (accessed on 12 November 2012).
8. Owen O'Donnell, Eddy van Doorslaer, Ravi P. Rannan-Eliya, Aparnaa Somanathan, Shiva Raj Adhikari, Deni Harbianto, Charu C. Garg, Piya Hanvoravongchai, Mohammed N. Huq, Anup Karan, and *et al*. "The incidence of public spending on healthcare: Comparative evidence from Asia." *The World Bank Economic Review* 21 (2007): 93–123.
9. Obinna Onwujekwe, Kara Hanson, and Benjamin Uzochukwu. "Are the poor differentially benefiting from provision of priority public health services? A benefit incidence analysis in Nigeria." *International Journal for Equity in Health* 11 (2012): 1–12.
10. Adam Wagstaff. "Benefit-incidence analysis: Are government health expenditures more pro-rich than we think? " *Health Economics* 21 (2012): 351–66.
11. Eddy Van Doorslaer, Owen O'Donnell, Ravi P. Rannan-Eliya, Aparnaa Somanathan, Shiva Raj Adhikari, Charu C. Garg, Deni Harbianto, Alejandro N. Herrin, Mohammed Nazmul Huq, Shamsia Ibragimova, and *et al*. "Effect of payments for health care on poverty estimates in 11 countries in Asia: An analysis of household survey data." *The Lancet* 368 (2006): 1357–64.

12. Ahmed Shoukry Rashad, and Mesbah Fathy Sharaf. "Catastrophic and Impoverishing Effects of Out-of-Pocket Health Expenditure: New Evidence from Egypt." *American Journal of Economics* 5 (2015): 526–33.
13. Laura Anselmi, Mylene Lagarde, and Kara Hanson. "Equity in the allocation of public sector financial resources in low-and middle-income countries: A systematic literature review." *Health Policy and Planning* 30 (2014): czu034.
14. Adam Wagstaff, Marcel Bilger, Leander R. Buisman, and Caryn Bredenkamp. "Who benefits from government health spending and why? A global assessment." 2014. Available online: http://papers.ssrn.com/sol3/Papers.cfm?abstract_id=2500586 (accessed on 10 February 2015).
15. James Akazili, Bertha Garshong, Moses Aikins, John Gyapong, and Di McIntyre. "Progressivity of health care financing and incidence of service benefits in Ghana." *Health Policy and Planning* 27 (2012): i13–22.
16. Ronelle Burger, Caryn Bredenkamp, Christelle Grobler, and Servaas van der Berg. "Have public health spending and access in South Africa become more equitable since the end of apartheid?" *Development Southern Africa* 29 (2012): 681–703.
17. Supon Limwattananon, Viroj Tangcharoensathien, Kanjana Tisayaticom, Tawekiat Boonyapaisarncharoen, and Phusit Prakongsai. "Why has the Universal Coverage Scheme in Thailand achieved a pro-poor public subsidy for health care?" *BMC Public Health* 12 (2012): S6.
18. Mingsheng Chen, Guixia Fang, Lidan Wang, Zhonghua Wang, Yuxin Zhao, and Lei Si. "Who Benefits from Government Healthcare Subsidies? An Assessment of the Equity of Healthcare Benefits Distribution in China." *PLoS ONE* 10 (2015): e0119840.
19. Laura Anselmi, Mylène Lagarde, and Kara Hanson. "Going beyond horizontal equity: An analysis of health expenditure allocation across geographic areas in Mozambique." *Social Science & Medicine* 130 (2015): 216–24.
20. Ravi P. Rannan-Eliya, Claudia Blanco-Vidal, and A. K. Nandakumar. *The Distribution of Health Care Resources in Egypt: Implications for Equity*. Boston: Harvard School of Public Health, 2000.
21. Sherine Shawky. "Could the employment-based targeting approach serve Egypt in moving towards a social health insurance model?" *Eastern Mediterranean Health Journal* 16 (2010): 663.
22. Fatma El Zanaty, and Ann Way. "Egypt Demographic and Health Survey 2008." 2009. Available online: http://dhsprogram.com/pubs/pdf/fr220/fr220.pdf (accessed on 5 December 2014).
23. Sharon Nakhimovsky, Douglas Glandon, Nadwa Rafeh, and Nagwan Hassan. "Egypt National Health Accounts: 2008/09." 2011. Available online: http://pdf.usaid.gov/pdf_docs/pnadz604.pdf (accessed on 10 September 2014).
24. Di McIntyre, and John E. Ataguba. "How to do (or not to do) ... a benefit incidence analysis." *Health Policy and Planning* 26 (2011): 174–82.
25. Owen O'Donnell. "Access to health care in developing countries: Breaking down demand side barriers." *Cadernos de Saúde Pública* 23 (2007): 2820–34.

26. World Health Organization. *The World Health Report 2008: Primary Health Care Now More Than Ever*. Geneva: World Health Organization, 2008.
27. Benjamin Loevinsohn, and April Harding. "Buying results? Contracting for health service delivery in developing countries." *The Lancet* 366 (2005): 676–81.
28. A. Venkat Raman, and James Warner Björkman. *Public-Private Partnerships in Health Care in India: Lessons for Developing Countries*. London: Routledge, 2008.
29. Ann Levin, and Miloud Kaddar. "Role of the private sector in the provision of immunization services in low-and middle-income countries." *Health Policy and Planning* 26 (2011): i4–12.

The Effectiveness of Healthy Community Approaches on Positive Health Outcomes in Canada and the United States

Hazel Williams-Roberts, Bonnie Jeffery, Shanthi Johnson and Nazeem Muhajarine

Abstract: Healthy community approaches encompass a diverse group of population based strategies and interventions that create supportive environments, foster community behavior change and improve health. This systematic review examined the effectiveness of ten most common healthy community approaches (Healthy Cities/Communities, Smart Growth, Child Friendly Cities, Safe Routes to Schools, Safe Communities, Active Living Communities, Livable Communities, Social Cities, Age-Friendly Cities, and Dementia Friendly Cities) on positive health outcomes. Empirical studies were identified through a search of the academic and grey literature for the period 2000–2014. Of the 231 articles retrieved, 26 met the inclusion criteria with four receiving moderate quality ratings and 22 poor ratings using the Effective Public Health Practice Project Quality Assessment Tool. The majority of studies evaluated Safe Routes to School Programs and reported positive associations with students' active commute patterns. Fewer studies assessed benefits of Smart Growth, Safe Communities, Active Living Communities and Age-Friendly Cities. The remaining approaches were relatively unexplored in terms of their health benefits however focused on conceptual frameworks and collaborative processes. More robust studies with longer follow-up duration are needed. Priority should be given to evaluation of healthy community projects to show their effectiveness within the population health context.

Reprinted from *Soc. Sci.* Cite as: Williams-Roberts, H.; Jeffery, B.; Johnson, S.; Muhajarine, N. The Effectiveness of Healthy Community Approaches on Positive Health Outcomes in Canada and the United States. *Soc. Sci.* **2016**, *5*, 3.

1. Introduction

Health is shaped by the daily conditions in which we are born, live, work, play and age [1]. These social determinants of health engender differential exposures and vulnerability to health damaging conditions and influence an individual's opportunities to live a healthy life. This is the fundamental basis for socioecological models that frame health as the confluence of multiple factors that operate in a nested genetic, biological, behavioral, social and environmental context [2]. Consequently, interventions that seek to improve health outcomes must target multiple levels and engage multisectoral partners to create the supportive conditions that foster healthy choices across settings and throughout the lifecycle.

Healthy community interventions offer a local societal response to address common threats to population health. The term "healthy communities", originally coined in Canada in the 1980s, refer to communities that employed health promotion and community development strategies to address multiple determinants of health [3].

The built and social environment sometimes limit the resources available to individuals and communities and make it difficult to adopt and maintain healthy behaviors [4]. Community efforts to promote health often target one or both of these domains. The general discourse on this subject is broad and without any specific model that cuts across all approaches. A community's vision for health is unique and can be pursued through multiple strategies according to their needs, assets and resources. In this article, the term healthy community approach was operationalized as deliberate efforts to improve health at the local/community level. The scope of the review was focused on health promoting strategies and interventions that target the social and physical environment, reflecting the importance of non-medical determinants in health.

The Healthy Communities Unit of the Public Health Agency of Canada commissioned this review and set out to inform their work priorities by understanding which approaches were effective in promoting the health of communities. As a result of their considerable experience with some approaches such as Age Friendly Cities, there was particular interest in approaches that target the social environment, while all the same recognizing the emerging emphasis in the literature on changing the built environment. Ten most common approaches including Healthy Cities/Healthy Communities, Smart Growth Planning, Child Friendly Cities, Safe Routes to Schools, Safe Communities, Active Living Communities, Livable Communities, Social Cities, Age-Friendly Cities, and Dementia Friendly Cities were selected for further examination. These were selected to be representative of healthy community approaches and reflect a balanced focus on the social and built environment in concert with the current understanding of determinants of health. The majority of these initiatives have global momentum that supports national efforts, are grounded in the mandate of a coordinating entity and employ multiple strategies (e.g., policies, services and structures) in various settings to achieve the objectives. There is considerable overlap in the goals and objectives with some initiatives nested within the priority areas of broader approaches. Table 1 describes the key elements of each approach. In this review each initiative has been presented independently although at the local level, these initiatives may be implemented synergistically, or as part of integrated efforts to improve health and wellbeing of communities.

There has been growing interest in the implementation of healthy community approaches with concomitant investment of public and private resources. One example is provided by the federal funding commitment of $612 million US dollars to support Safe Routes to School (SRTS) Programs in the United States [15,16]. The Robert Wood Johnson Foundation has also provided several grants in the sum of US$200,000 to support Active Living by Design (ALbD) projects [17]. With limited resources to support project implementation, it is important to determine which approaches have demonstrated benefits for whom and under what circumstances. Despite active research in some areas, evidence of effectiveness is still relatively scarce. Few reviews have explored selected approaches including SRTS and Safe Communities; however, note the absence of evidence of program impact on health outcomes [18,19]. The Cochrane systematic review of the effectiveness of WHO Safe Communities model excluded the few identified studies from the US because no injury outcomes were assessed [19]. To the best of our knowledge, this group of approaches have not previously been examined collectively nor with a specific geographical focus.

The purpose of this review was to evaluate the evidence for the effectiveness of the ten most common healthy community approaches on positive health outcomes in Canada and the United States. This bridges a gap in the literature about what is effective and informs future priorities for research to strengthen the evidence base. The heterogeneity of interventions, study designs and outcomes as well as the small number of studies identified precluded meta-analysis. A qualitative approach with narrative synthesis of the available evidence is presented.

Table 1. Description of healthy community approaches.

Healthy Community Approaches	Target population	Description
Healthy Cities	Whole populations	World Health Organization (WHO) initiative established in 1986 that seeks to protect health and support sustainable development. The basic features are community participation and empowerment, intersectoral collaboration, equity and action to address the social determinants of health [5].
Child Friendly Cities	Children	Launched in 1996, this global movement supported by United Nations Children's Fund (UNICEF) promotes children's rights to the highest quality of life. The nine elements include children's participation in issues that involve them, child friendly legal framework, children's rights strategy, child rights unit, child impact assessment, budget to support children's activities, children's national report, advocacy for children's rights and children's ombudsman or commissioner [6].

Table 1. *Cont.*

Healthy Community Approaches	Target population	Description
Smart Growth Planning	Whole populations	An approach, first launched in 1995, to land use planning and development that supports health, economic growth and prioritizes conservation. The ten fundamental principles include: mixed land use, promoting compact building design, providing a range of housing options, fostering attractive communities with a strong sense of place, preservation of open spaces, development of existing communities, variety of transportation choices, encouraging fair and cost effective development and supporting community collaboration in development [7].
Safe Routes to School	Children in school settings	The US national program that uses multiple modalities including education, engineering improvements, enforcement and encouragement to increase student active travel [8]. Although activities occurred as early as 1997 in the US, the National Program Safe Routes to School Program was established by federal legislation in 2005.
Safe Communities	Whole populations	A global initiative supported by WHO that engages communities to promote safety and injury prevention. Multiple global networks have been established and provide accreditation to committed communities who satisfy the designated criteria [9]. The concept was introduced as a policy initiative in Sweden in 1989.
Active Living Communities	Whole populations in selected communities	A movement that is dedicated to increasing opportunities for population physical activity. Some projects may include other components such as Safe Routes to School or Smart Growth [10]. Active Living by Design (ALbD) was at the forefront of the movement and was launched in 2002.
Livable Communities	Whole populations	Livable communities embody multiple factors that contribute to good quality of life such as recreational and educational opportunities, attractive built and natural environment, social stability and economic prosperity [11]. Programs have been implemented by various partners for more than 25 years.
Social Cities	Whole Populations	A social city fosters social connectedness of its residents and improves the social architecture to strengthen these relationships [12]. The concept has been growing in popularity since 2009.
Age-Friendly Cities	Elderly population	Global Initiative that promotes active aging of older residents and increases opportunities for their social participation and security. The movement builds on the 2002 Policy Framework for Active Aging and considers key domains of the social and physical environment that need to be optimized to enhance the quality of life of older persons. These include the outdoor spaces and buildings, transportation, housing, social participation, respect and social inclusion, civic participation and employment, communication and information, community support and health [13].
Dementia Friendly Cities	Persons living with dementia and their care givers	This initiative is supported by the Alzheimer's Society and seeks to improve inclusion and quality of life of people living with dementia [14]. It has been gaining momentum especially in the United Kingdom since 2012.

2. Methods

2.1. Data Sources and Search Strategy

The studies included in this review were identified through a systematic search of the academic and grey literature. Peer reviewed publications were searched in selected electronic databases including PubMed, Medline, Cumulative Index to Nursing and Allied Health Literature (CINAHL), Scopus and the Cochrane Library. The reference lists of all included papers were examined for additional articles not discovered through the primary search.

Google Scholar was used to search the web based literature to identify additional articles of relevance such as dissertations, reports, conference presentations and abstracts. A search of the grey literature focused on initiative specific websites (e.g., Child Friendly Cities, Safe Communities Canada, Active and Safe Routes to School) and websites of agencies coordinating the respective approaches (e.g., UNICEF, World Health Organization). Other relevant resources consulted included the Best Practices Portal, Centers for Disease Control (CDC) Community Interventions Evidence Database, the National Transportation Library (NTL), the McMaster University's General Database of Public Health Interventions and the Effective Public Health Practice Policy Portal.

Three domains of search terms were identified: effectiveness, 'healthy community approaches' and country/geographical region. Specific terms used for the search were derived from the subject headings in MeSH list, free text and review studies related to the selected approaches. Search strategies were tailored for each approach and adapted for different databases. An example of the search strategy used for Safe Routes to School approach is shown in Appendix. Searches were limited to papers published in the English language during the period January 2000 to December 2014. A diverse range of studies with both experimental and observational study designs were included. This allowed for consideration of evidence from interventions that could not be randomized for practical or ethical reasons. Systematic reviews were excluded as empirical research was thought to offer the best available quality of evidence.

2.2. Selection and Review Process

Studies were screened initially using titles and abstracts. All articles that were potentially relevant were subjected to a detailed assessment. Studies selected were required to meet the following inclusion criteria: (1) explicitly reference an intervention based on one of the ten healthy community approaches; (2) measure at least one health outcome (morbidity, mortality or intermediary outcomes); and (3) conducted in North America (limited to Canada and United States). The following exclusion criteria were applied to the search results: (1) the article was an opinion, editorial, audit or review; (2) it included only a description of an approach but no assessment of its impact on health outcomes; and (3) employed only qualitative methods. Any disagreements about inclusion of studies were resolved through consensus of the authors. Relevant data was extracted from the articles including descriptive information; indicators of quality and measures of effectiveness. The quality of the evidence was assessed using the Effective Public Health Practice Project (EPHPP) Quality Assessment Tool for quantitative studies. The tool and accompanying dictionary are available at http://www.ephpp.ca [20]. The EPHPP examines six methodological dimensions: selection bias, study design, confounders, blinding, data collection methods, withdrawals and dropouts. A rating of strong, moderate or weak was assigned for each of the study components and then a global rating was calculated.

3. Results and Discussion

The search identified 1415 potential articles among the various sources. From these papers, 231 were assessed for eligibility based on full text review. Twenty six articles were selected and subsequently underwent quality assessment. There were no studies that received a methodologically strong rating, four were of moderate quality and 22 were assessed as weak. The main reasons for weak ratings included selection bias, failure to control for confounding and high attrition. A flow diagram of the search results is illustrated in Figure 1.

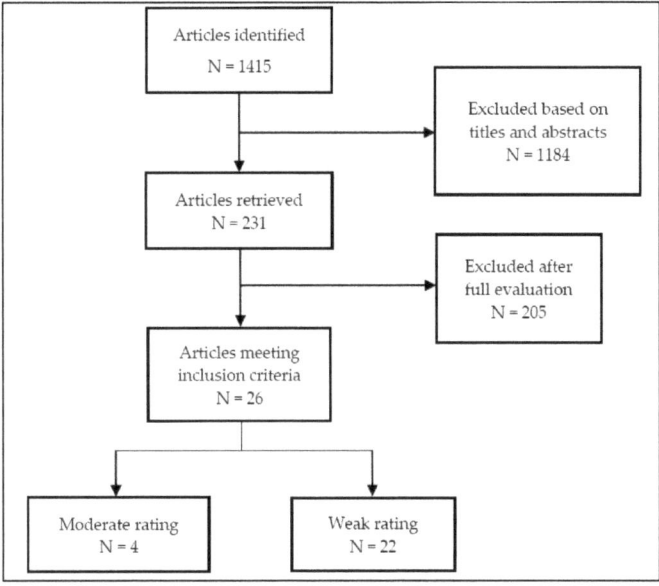

Figure 1. Summary of search and selection process for identification of relevant studies.

3.1. Safe Routes to School

The majority of studies identified were related to evaluation of Safe Routes to School Programs (SRTS) in the United States (Table 2). In terms of study quality assessed using the EPHPP tool, most studies were assessed as weak based on methodological limitations. Two studies that examined the impact of Walking School Bus (WSB) interventions received moderate ratings. The earlier of the two studies assessed the short and long term effects on student travel in a low income minority population [21]. Another pilot study by Mendoza and colleagues employed a cluster randomized controlled trial to investigate the impact of a five week WSB intervention on rates of active commuting and physical activity levels [22]. Most studies employed multifaceted interventions that included education, traffic enforcement and engineering improvements however a few studies utilized only one strategy (commonly walking school bus) to influence active modes of school transportation [21–34]. Consistent with the goal of increasing rates of children's active transportation to and from school, most studies focused on reporting intermediary outcomes such as travel behavior and attitudes. Only two studies also incorporated objective measures of physical activity to corroborate the results [21,34].

While the overwhelming emphasis of study outcomes focused on rates of active travel, five articles attempted to estimate the safety benefits that accrue from SRTS programs [35–39]. Di Maggio and Li found that annual rates of pedestrian injuries in children aged 5–19 years decreased in census tracts with SRTS improvements when compared to those census tracts without projects [35]. Two other studies reported a change in the number of collisions involving school aged children over baseline for intervention and control/comparison sites [36,37]. However, neither study could conclusively confirm the safety effects of Safe Routes to School Programs because of limitations inherent in the study design and lack of data on other correlates of collisions that may offer alternative explanations for the results. Another recent study by Ragland *et al.* also found a significant reduction in collisions involving pedestrians of all ages within 250 feet of countermeasure buffer zones [38]. Although a decrease in collisions also occurred among pedestrians aged 5 to 18 years, it was not statistically significant.

Table 2. Summary of Quality Assessment of Studies using Effective Public Health Practice Project Tool (EPHPP).

Author/Date	Selection Bias	Study Design	Confounders	Blinding	Data Collection Methods	Withdrawals/ Drop outs	Global Rating
Safe Routes to School							
Mendoza et al., 2009 [21]	Moderate	Moderate	Weak	N/A	Strong	Moderate	Moderate
Mendoza et al., 2011 [22]	Weak	Moderate	Weak	Moderate	Strong	Weak	Weak
Boarnet et al., 2005 [23]	Weak	Weak	Weak	Moderate	Weak	Moderate	Weak
Cooper et al., 2010 [24]	Weak	Moderate	Weak	Moderate	Strong	Weak	Weak
Buliung et al., 2011 [25]	Weak	Weak	Weak	Moderate	Weak	Weak	Weak
Mammen et al., 2014 [26]	Weak	Moderate	Moderate	N/A	Strong	Weak	Weak
Henderson et al.2013 [27]	Weak	Moderate	Weak	Moderate	Weak	Weak	Weak
McDonald et al., 2013 [28]	Weak	Moderate	Moderate	Moderate	Strong	Moderate	Weak
McDonald et al., 2014 [29]	Weak	Weak	Strong	Moderate	Strong	Weak	Weak
McDonald et al., 2013 [28]	Weak	Moderate	Moderate	Moderate	Strong	Weak	Weak
Moudon et al., 2012 [30]	Weak	Weak	Moderate	N/A	Weak	Strong	Weak
Staunton et al., 2003 [31]	Weak	Weak	Weak	N/A	Moderate	Weak	Weak
Buckley et al., 2013 [32]	Weak	Moderate	Weak	Moderate	Weak	Weak	Weak
Johnson et al., 2006 [33]	Weak	Moderate	Weak	Weak	Moderate	Weak	Weak
Sayers et al., 2012 [34]	Weak	Weak	Strong	Weak	Moderate	Weak	Weak
Di Maggio et al., 2013 [35]	Moderate	Moderate	Weak	Moderate	Moderate	Moderate	Moderate
Blomberg et al.,2008 [36]	Moderate	Weak	Weak	Moderate	Weak	Moderate	Weak
Orenstein et al., 2007 [37]	Moderate	Weak	Weak	N/A	Weak	Moderate	Weak
Ragland et al., 2014 [38]	Weak	Weak	Weak	Moderate	Strong	Weak	Weak
Mendoza et al., 2012 [39]	Weak	Strong	Moderate	Moderate	Strong	Weak	Weak
Active living communities							
Chomitz, 2012 [40]	Moderate	Moderate	Strong	Weak	Strong	Moderate	Moderate
TenBrink et al., 2009 [41]	Weak	Weak	Weak	Weak	Weak	Weak	Weak
Sayers et al., 2012 [42]	Weak	Weak	Weak	Weak	Moderate	Moderate	Weak
Safe communities							
Istre et al., 2011 [43]	Weak	Moderate	Weak	Weak	Weak	Moderate	Weak
Smart growth planning							
Dunton et al., 2011 [44]	Weak	Moderate	Weak	Moderate	Moderate	Strong	Weak
Age-friendly cities							
Lehning et al., 2012 [45]	Strong	Weak	Strong	Weak	Strong	Moderate	Weak
Menec and Nowicki, 2014 [46]	Weak	Weak	Strong	Weak	Moderate	Moderate	Weak

Mendoza and colleagues also assessed the impact of a brief WSB intervention on pedestrian safety behaviors [39]. They found that children at intervention schools were more likely to cross at the corner or crosswalk at intersections (OR = 5.01, 95% CI 2.79–8.99) although fewer children stopped at the curb compared to children in control schools (OR = 0.21, 95% CI 0.15–0.31). Although a randomized control trial, the brief duration of the intervention limits conclusions about sustainability of behavior change. Additionally, observations were made of all children at intersections whether or not they were study participants. This would tend to underestimate any effects. Future studies that gather longitudinal data on WSB study participants would be more useful to confirm these results.

In Canada, School Travel Planning (STP) is the vehicle to promote Active Safe Routes to Schools Programs (ASRTS) by engaging stakeholders to develop and implement action plans that are sustainable at the local level. There were two studies that explored the effect of STP interventions on student active school travel [25,26]. Buliung and colleagues conducted the first pilot study of twelve schools across four Canadian provinces [25]. Over a two year period, the proportion of children (grades K—8) who used active modes of transportation for their daily school commute was monitored. There was a slight increase in the percentage of children who use active modes of travel from 43.8% at baseline to 45.9% at follow up. Parental attitudes were also more supportive of active modes of transportation in pilot schools.

A larger study consisting of 106 public elementary schools was implemented in 2010 across nine Canadian provinces [26]. Data was only available for 53 schools. There was no significant increase in active school travel after a year. In multivariable models, only season of data collection predicted a decrease in active travel in the morning. More research is needed to confirm the efficacy of STP interventions. Variation in mode change was noted between schools which suggests that other contextual factors may be important for success. Furthermore, a year may not have been adequate to demonstrate benefits of the intervention given the varied needs and heterogeneity of interventions.

There is a growing body of literature about the impact of Safe Routes to School (SRTS) programs fueled by the need to evaluate SRTS projects that received US federal funding through the Safe Accountable Flexible Efficient Transportation Equity Act: A Legacy for Users (SAFETEA-LU), often for infrastructural projects. The available evidence to support an effect of Safe Routes to School Programs on rates of active commute shows a consistent positive association although the strength of impact is generally weak. There is less evidence to support safety benefits of programs although studies suggest a reduction in morbidity from injuries. Only a few studies employ robust designs that address common threats to internal validity such as selection bias, include objective measures of health outcomes and adjust for potential confounding factors in multivariable analyses. Longer duration of follow up is also needed to demonstrate the sustainability of efforts. Future studies must address these limitations in order to strengthen the evidence base related to effectiveness of these interventions.

Among other healthy community approaches included in this review, there was a paucity of evidence to support a positive impact on health outcomes. There were relatively few studies identified with three studies related to Active Living Communities [40–42]; one each for Safe communities [43] and Smart growth [44] and two related to Age Friendly Cities [45,46]. While various study designs were employed, none were randomized controlled trials. The assessment of methodological quality also revealed low ratings as a result of selection bias, less rigorous study designs and analytic methods. The characteristics of various studies are reported in narrative format in Table 3 where information is provided about study design, interventions and outcomes.

Table 3. Summary of evidence for effectiveness of interventions.

Study	Outcomes
Safe Routes to School	
Mendoza *et al.*, 2009 [21] <ul><li>*Study design:* Quasi-experimental design (pre-post intervention with control group)</li><li>*Sample:* 653 (baseline) 643 (follow up)</li><li>*Study population:* Ethnically diverse children (ages 5–11 years) attending three elementary public schools in Seattle.</li><li>*Approach:* This study evaluates the impact of a Walking School Bus intervention in 3 urban Seattle public schools on patterns of active travel.</li></ul>	The proportion of children who walked to intervention (20% ± 2%) and control schools (15% ± 2%) was similar at baseline. At 12 month follow up, a higher proportion of children walked to intervention schools (25% ± 2%) compared to control schools (7% ± 1%, $p = 0.001$).
Mendoza *et al.*, 2011 [22] <ul><li>*Study design:* Cluster randomized controlled trial.</li><li>*Sample:* 149 children</li><li>*Study population:* 4th graders in 8 schools in Houston, Texas.</li><li>*Approach:* This pilot study examined the impact of a walking school bus intervention on children's physical activity levels and rates of active school travel</li></ul>	Weekly percent active commuting increased in the intervention group, while a decrease was observed in the control group ($p < 0.0001$). Acculturation and parent outcome expectations were associated with a change in percent active commuting. In multivariable models predicting minutes of moderate to vigorous physical activity, children in the intervention group increased their minutes while a decline was observed in the participants in the control group ($p = 0.029$).
Boarnet *et al.*, 2005 [23] <ul><li>*Study design:* Cross sectional design</li><li>*Sample size:* 1244 parental surveys</li><li>*Study population:* Children in 3rd to 5th grades of 10 elementary schools.</li><li>*Approach:* The study evaluated the effect of California SRTS engineering and infrastructure improvement projects on children's active school commuting patterns in 10 elementary schools.</li></ul>	Among children who passed the project on the way to school, a greater proportion (15.4%) walked or bicycled more after the construction projects when compared to children who did not (4.3%) encounter the projects on the way to school ($p < 0.01$).

Table 3. *Cont.*

Study	Outcomes
Cooper *et al.*, 2010 [24] <ul><li>*Study design:* Quasi-experimental design (pre-post intervention)</li><li>*Sample size:* 846 (baseline), 470 (follow up)</li><li>*Study population:* Children in 10 elementary schools in low income communities across United States.</li><li>*Approach:* The study evaluated the impact of SRTS programs delivered by coordinators on students' active travel commute patterns.</li></ul>	Parental surveys reported modest increases in children walking to (29%) and from (26%) school over baseline. However student tallies showed marked variation with smaller increases (1 to 5%) in schools with paid coordinators and only one of the other six schools showed a clear increase (7% to 14%) in walking. In general, schools with paid coordinators had 50% more students walking in the morning and 45% in the afternoon than schools with volunteers.
Buliung *et al.*, 2011 [25] <ul><li>*Study design:* Quasi-experimental design (pre-post intervention without control group)</li><li>*Sample:* 1489 parental surveys</li><li>*Study population:* parents of children in 12 elementary schools spread across 4 Canadian provinces.</li><li>*Approach:* The pilot study assessed the efficacy of school travel planning as an approach to facilitate active travel among students.</li></ul>	Small increases occurred in rates of active transportation from 43.5% (baseline) to 45.9% (follow up). Higher rates (43.5%) of active travel occurred at afternoons compared to mornings (37.3%). Among household respondents, 13.3% indicated that the intervention "resulted in less driving".

Safe Routes to School

Study	Outcomes
Mammen *et al.*, 2014 [26] <ul><li>*Study design:* Quasi-experimental design (pre-post intervention without control group)</li><li>*Sample:* 53 schools across Canada</li><li>*Study population:* Children (grades K—8) in participating elementary schools</li><li>*Approach:* The study examined the effectiveness of STP in Canada on students' rates of active travel and identified predictors of mode change.</li></ul>	There was no increase over baseline in rates of active travel either in morning or afternoon after one year. Marked variation occurred in AST at the school level. The season of data collection predicted a decrease in AST in the morning ($p < 0.05$).
Henderson *et al.*, 2013 [27] <ul><li>*Study design:* Quasi-experimental design (pre-post intervention without control group)</li><li>*Sample:* 658 students</li><li>*Study population:* children and their parents from one elementary school in Atlanta.</li><li>*Approach:* The study assessed the impact of a multifaceted SRTS program in an elementary school in Atlanta over 2008–2010.</li></ul>	There was an increase in the rates of walking to school in the morning ($p < 0.0001$) during the intervention period however no significant change was observed for the afternoon commute. Parental perception about school support for active modes of transport and the health benefits ($0.01 < p < 0.001$) and enjoyment associated with active modes of transportation ($p < 0.0001$) also improved.

Table 3. *Cont.*

Study	Outcomes
McDonald *et al.*, 2013 [28] • *Study design:* Quasi-experimental design (pre-post intervention with control groups). • *Sample:* 1000–2300 students each year. • *Study population:* Children (K-8) attending 9 intervention and 5 comparison schools in the 4J school district of Oregon. • *Approach:* The study evaluated the impact of a SRTS program on walking and biking to school in Eugene, Oregon.	Regression models were used to estimate the marginal effects associated with walking or biking to school among the study population. Schools with more types of interventions had larger proportions of students who walked or biked to school. Programs that delivered education and encouragement components in addition to two other SRTS interventions were associated with a 20 percentage point increase in walking and a small but non-significant increase in biking. Infrastructure improvement interventions had borderline significance which might have been related to late completion of these components in the program cycle. Provision of covered bike parking was associated with large increases in walking (19 percentage points) and biking (11 percentage points). The Boltage intervention produced small increases in walking (5 percentage points) and biking (4 percentage points).
McDonald *et al.*, 2014 [29] • *Study design:* Cross sectional design • *Sample:* School travel and program data analyzed from 801 schools in four US States • *Study population:* School travel mode data for the period 2007–2012 from schools in 4 US states • *Approach:* The study assessed the impact of SRTS programs on students' active travel by comparing schools with and without SRTS programs	Fractional logit models were used to estimate the marginal effects of the presence and number of years of SRTS interventions on walking and bicycling. Rates of active travel increased with each year of participation in SRTS programs. After five years, there was an absolute increase of 13 percentage points in the proportion of children who walked or biked. In multivariable models after adjustment for school and environmental characteristics, walking and bicycling rose by 1.1 percentage points for each year of participation in SRTS programs. The presence of an engineering component was associated with 3.3 percentage point increase in walking and bicycling. This was unrelated to the length of time that the improvement was in place. Smaller increases (0.9 percentage points) were associated with education and encouragement interventions.

Safe Routes to School

Study	Outcomes
Moudon *et al.*, 2012 [30] • *Study design:* Cross sectional design • *Sample:* Active travel data was available for 48 of the 569 SRTS projects. • *Study population:* The study utilized secondary data obtained pre and post implementation of SRTS projects to estimate the impact on student travel patterns. • *Approach:* This study assessed the impact of SRTS programs on children's active school travel in five US states.	There was a statistically significant increase in rates of active transport for all modes of transport in all states except for biking in Florida. Rates of walking increased more than cycling. Changes in rates of active transport were not correlated with any project, school or neighborhood characteristics.
Staunton *et al.*, 2003 [31] • *Study design:* Quasi-experimental design (pre-post intervention without control group) • *Sample:* 13 schools (6 in year 1 and 7 in year 2) • *Study population:* children in 15 elementary schools in Marin County, California • *Approach:* The study examined the impact of SRTS program on active travel of children to and from school.	There were marked increases in walking (64%), biking (114%) and carpooling (39% decrease in children arriving by car) over the two year period.

Table 3. *Cont.*

Study	Outcomes
Buckley *et al.* 2013 [32] • *Study design:* Quasi-experimental design (with pre, during and post event assessments with control group) • *Sample:* 475 students for fall event and 238 students for spring event. • *Study population:* Children and parents partiicpanting in designated 'Walk t oSchool Day events at two elementary schools in Moscow, Idaho • *Approach:* The study examined the impact of two Walk to School Day events on active school travel patterns in children at two elementary schools	The number of children who walked to school increased by 25% (19%–26%). During the same period, there was a decrease in the proportion of children walking to school at comparison sites. Direct observations of children at school crossings showed small improvements in street crossing safety over baseline however key desirable behaviors were present in less than 50% of all observed crossings.
Johnson *et al.*, 2006 [33] • *Study design:* Quasi-experimental design (pre-post intervention with control group) • *Sample:* 695 (baseline) 782 (follow up) • *Study population:* Children attending three elementary public schools in Seattle. • *Approach:* This study evaluates the impact of a Walking School Bus intervention in an inner city Seattle public schools on patterns of active travel.	The number of children who walked to school increased by 25% (19%–26%). During the same period, there was a decrease in the proportion of children walking to school at comparison sites. Direct observations of children at school crossings showed small improvements in street crossing safety over baseline however key desirable behaviors were present in less than 50% of all observed crossings.
Sayers *et al.*, 2012 [34] • *Study design:* Cross sectional design. • *Sample:* 77 (38 intervention, 39 comparison) • *Study population:* Children at three elementary schools. • *Approach:* The study examined the effect of a walking school bus intervention on physical activity in three elementary schools in Missouri.	There was no difference between the groups in physical activity levels ($p = 0.17$). The percentage of time spent in moderate to vigorous physical activity (MVPA) during the study was 38 (20.9 $\pm$ 6.9) for WSB participants and 39 (23.4 $\pm$ 8) in comparison group. In multivariable models, age was negatively associated with percentage of time spent in moderate to vigorous physical activity ($r = -0.79$, $p < 0.001$).

Safe Routes to School

Di Maggio and Li 2013 [35] • *Study design:* Time series analysis. • *Sample:* Authors compared age specific rates of pedestrian injuries in census tracts with and without SRTS interventions. • *Study population:* Study used crash data from the Department of Transportation from 2001–2010 and data related to the location of planned SRTS projects. • *Approach:* The study examined the impact of Safe Routes to School (SRTS) interventions on morbidity resulting from pedestrian injury in school aged children in New York City.	Annual pedestrian injuries declined over time however the most pronounced reduction (33% 95% CI 30–36) was observed among school aged children (5–19 years) compared to 14% (95% CI 12–16) among other age groups. Pedestrian injury rates among school aged children in census tracts with SRTS interventions decreased between the pre-intervention and post intervention periods as well as during school travel hours (8 to 4.4 injuries per 10,000 persons). These observations were not apparent in census tracts without SRTS interventions.

Table 3. *Cont.*

Study	Outcomes
Blomberg *et al.* 2008 [36] • *Study design*: Time series analysis based on secondary data • *Sample*: SRTS data for 130 legacy programs, state crash data from 1996 to current year • *Study population*: • *Approach*: To examine the safety effects of implementing legacy SRTS programs in three states with the largest number of SRTS programs	There was a general decline in pedestrian and bicycling collison sover time. Marked reductions occurred for children 4 to 12 yeats served by SRTS focus sites when compared to state wide collisons, although the differences were not statistically significant.
Orenstein *et al.*, 2007 [37] • *Study design:* Time series analysis using secondary data. • *Sample:* 125 SRTS programs and collision data from 1998–2005. • *Study population:* The analysis was based on national data for injuries and fatalities that resulted from collisions and SRTS project data. • *Approach:* This study was commissioned to assess the safety impact of SRTS programs in California.	The authors compared the change in injuries involving school aged children (5 to 18 years) pre and post SRTS construction projects for intervention and control sites in California. There was a general decline in the number of injuries between 1998 and 2005 with a similar percentage reduction in the annual number of injuries for both SRTS (13%) and non SRTS sites (15%). However when the changes in mobility patterns were accounted for, it was estimated that safety benefits ranged from no net change to a decrease of 49% in collisions among students at SRTS sites.
Ragland *et al.*, 2014 [38] • *Study design:* Cross sectional design • *Sample:* 47 schools, mobility analysis from 1999 parental surveys received from 8 schools. • *Study population:* Schools in California that had implemented SRTS infrastructural improvements. • *Approach:* The study assessed the long term impact of SRTS funded infrastructural improvements on safety and walking and bicycling to school.	In pedestrians ages 8 to 18 years there was a 50% reduction in collisions in the treatment area (within 250 feet of the countermeasure buffer zones). Although effect not statistically significant. Among pedestrians of all ages, there was a statistically significant 75% reduction of collisions in the treated areas compared to control areas. In the mobility analysis, living within 250 feet of the SRTS project improvement was associated with an increased probability of walking to school.
Mendoza *et al.*, 2012 [39] • *Study design:* Cluster randomized controlled trial (4 intervention, 4 control schools) • *Sample:* 1252 (pre) 2548 (post) pedestrian observations at intersections. • *Study population:* 4th grade elementary school children in 8 schools in Houston school district. • *Approach:* The study assessed the impact of WSB intervention on child pedestrian safety behaviors at street intersections.	Compared to children at control schools, children at intervention schools has five times higher odds of crossing at crosswalk or corner (95% CI 2.79–8.99, $p < 0.01$) however also had five fold lower odds of stopping at the curb 95% CI 0.15–0.31, $p < 0.01$). Parent perception of neighborhood safety and number of traffic lanes were not associated with pedestrian safety outcomes in mixed models ($p > 0.05$).

Table 3. *Cont.*

Study	Outcomes
Active Living Communities	
Chomitz *et al.*, 2012 [40] <ul><li>*Study design:* Quasi-experimental design (pre-post intervention with control group)</li><li>*Sample:* intervention city—1081 (pre) and 644 (post); comparison city—608 (post)</li><li>*Study population:* Non-institutionalized adults over 18 years, children in targeted middle and high schools.</li><li>*Approach:* The study assessed the effectiveness of an Active Living by Design project in Somerville Massachusetts on physical activity levels</li></ul>	Adults in the intervention city were more likely than those in the comparison city to report meeting recommended physical activity guidelines (OR = 1.10, 95% CI 1.04–1.17). No differences were found in meeting the recommended physical activity guidelines among of children in both cities in adjusted analyses [middle school OR 1.06 (95% CI 0.78–1.45); high school OR 1.24 95% CI 0.98–1.58).
TenBrink *et al.*, 2009 [41] <ul><li>*Study design:* Quasi-experimental design (pre-post without control group)</li><li>*Sample:* An annual transportation survey conducted in 15 locations over a one week period provided data on pedestrian and cycling patters. Walking audits and employee surveys were used in the work place initiative.</li><li>*Study population:* Children in targeted schools, general population.</li><li>*Approach:* The study assessed the effects on travel behavior of an Active Living by Design project in Michigan.</li></ul>	The number of students who walked to school (5%–15% increase) and participation in sentinel events such as Walk to School Day and Smart Commute Day increased during the project. Participation in Smart Commute Day increased from 165 (2004) to 520 persons (2008). Walk to school day participants increased from 600 in 2003 to 1200 in 2008.
Sayers *et al.*, 2012 [42] <ul><li>*Study design:* Time series analysis</li><li>*Sample:* Quarterly assessments on five consecutive days at designated intersections each year of project.</li><li>*Study population:* Data based on seasonal direct observations of pedestrians and cyclists at four key intersections in Columbia.</li><li>*Approach:* The study examined the effects of a multifaceted intervention on rates of active travel in the community over a three year period.</li></ul>	Pedestrian and cyclists counts increased from 2007 to 2009 particularly in the latter part (July and October) of 2009. Repeated measures ANOVA showed a statistically significant effect of year ($p = 0.01$), season ($p < 0.001$) and interaction of year and season ($p = 0.05$). Survey data indicated increased awareness of ALbD programming through media and advertisements in 2008 compared to 2003 (63% of respondents, N = 813).
Safe Communities	
Istre *et al.*, 2011 [43] <ul><li>*Study design:* Quasi-experimental design (pre-post intervention with control group)</li><li>*Sample:* 9483 observations (5743 observations among children in the target communities).</li><li>*Study Population:* Data based on pre and post assessments of restraint use in motor vehicles at 34 sites in target and comparison communities.</li><li>*Approach:* The study sought to measure the effect of a WHO Safe community model approach on the use of child restraints among children 0–8 years in motor vehicles in Texas</li></ul>	In multivariable analyses, child restraint use (OR = 1.6 95% CI 1.2–2.2), drivers who were wearing a seatbelt (OR = 2.2 95% CI 1.5–3.2) and children riding in the back seat (OR = 1.3 95% CI 1.0–1.6) increased significantly over baseline for target communities compared to communities that did not receive the intervention.

Table 3. *Cont.*

Study	Outcomes
Smart Growth Planning	
Dunton *et al.*, 2012 [44] • *Study design:* Quasi-experimental study (pre-post intervention with control group). • *Sample:* 94 (48 intervention, 46 control) children • *Study population:* Children (9–13 years) who recently moved to smart growth community or who lived in neighboring community • *Approach:* This study explored the effect of smart growth communities on children's physical activity levels and whether the physical activity context differed over time compared to children in non-smart growth communities.	Children in smart growth communities engaged in a greater proportion of physical activity bouts a few blocks from home ($p < 0.001$) and travelled more by walking ($p < 0.011$) than children in control communities. Over time, social context of physical activity did not change for either group however children in smart growth communities were more likely to report decreased physical activity indoors and an increase in outdoor locations with no traffic ($p = 0.036$). There was a greater increase in six month daily moderate to vigorous physical activity among children in intervention communities however it was not statistically significant ($p = 0.10$).
Age-Friendly Cities	
Lehning *et al.*, 2012 [45] • *Study design:* Cross sectional design • *Sample:* 1386 persons • *Study population:* Non-institutionalized persons aged 60 years or older who resided in Detroit. • *Approach:* This study assessed the relationship between age-friendly environments and self-rated health among a sample of older adults in Detroit, Michigan.	In adjusted multivariable analyses, significant predictors of better self-rated health included access to health care ($p < 0.01$), social support ($p < 0.01$) and community engagement ($p < 0.01$) while neighborhood problems were associated with poorer self-rated health ($p < 0.01$). Addition of age-friendly environment characteristics weakened the association between self-rated health and three health measures (two functional limitations and chronic conditions) although still significant $p < 0.001$. Education and income variables were no longer significant when age-friendly characteristics were included in the model.
Menec and Nowicki, 2014 [46] • *Study design:* Cross sectional design • *Sample:* 593 individuals who completed an age-friendly survey. • *Study population:* Data were analyzed from a subset of 29 communities that completed a needs assessment as part of the Manitoba Age Friendly Initiative. • *Approach:* This study assessed the relationship between age-friendly characteristics of communities and residents' life satisfaction and self-perceived health in rural Manitoba	Higher Age-Friendly ratings were associated with greater life satisfaction ($p < 0.0001$) and self-perceived health (<0.01). In multivariable analyses among seniors, the Age-Friendly Index as well as five of the seven domains was associated with life satisfaction. Community support and health services were not associated with any health outcomes. Self-perceived health was associated with fewer age-friendly domains including physical environment, housing, social environment and transportation options. These results differed for younger respondents as age friendliness was not associated with self-perceived health and life satisfaction was only associated with health services/community support and opportunities for participation ($p < 0.05$).

3.2. Active Living Communities

Active Living Communities increase the opportunities for physical activity through the creation of supportive policies and infrastructure that foster active modes of commuting [47]. References to "active living" are common in the literature however a formal, universal definition is difficult to find. The most organized efforts to create a shared vision and operationalize the active community living concept have come from the Robert Wood Johnson Foundation in the United States. In 2003, the Robert Wood Johnson Foundation approved 25 grants to US communities to implement Active Living by Design (ALbD) Projects. These five year grants supported projects to promote physical activity by employing a Community Action Model with five components namely preparation, promotion, programs, policy influences and physical projects. Using this approach, communities assess their needs and devise unique solutions to transform local environments to foster opportunities for increased physical activity [17].

The ALbD Project evaluations in Massachusetts [40], Michigan [41] and Missouri [42] reported an increase in the number of persons using active modes of transportation over the study period; however, methodological limitations in these studies limit causal attribution of any effects solely to the project's influence. Project reports emphasize the changing community dynamics, rich partnerships and community empowerment that occur with project implementation as key achievements over health outcomes. More research is needed that focuses on measuring the effect of interventions on health outcomes in order to justify future investments in Active Living Initiatives.

3.3. Age-Friendly Cities

The review identified several narrative accounts of process evaluations of Age-Friendly Initiatives [48–51]. Despite this finding, there is a gap in knowledge about the holistic impact of Age-Friendly Initiatives on outcomes in the lives of older persons. The disparate results of the two studies suggest that further empirical evidence is needed that employs standardized definitions of age-friendly environments across diverse settings and health outcomes [45,46].

Cognizant of the need to update the monitoring and evaluation framework for the Age-Friendly Initiative to capture process as well as outcomes, the World Health Organization began work in 2012 to develop core indicators that would meet these expectations [52]. The proposed core indicators will retain the emphasis on tracking the progress towards the achievement of age-friendly environments however will include a few distal long term outcomes that reflect improved health and quality of life of older persons. This will pave the way for future project impact evaluations that report health outcomes.

3.4. Safe Communities

Safe Communities is an approach to injury prevention and safety promotion that embraces interventions at the community level [53]. The initiative advocates for multisectoral cooperation to devise local solutions to community safety concerns. Communities that satisfy established benchmark criteria receive the safe community designation. Evaluation frameworks emphasize the achievement of milestones in the planning process such as establishment of coordination structures, community assessment, plan development and mobilization of funding [54]. While discrete health outcomes may be measured (e.g., road traffic accidents, child mortality from unintentional injuries) in specific projects, the commitment is often to the process and creation of supportive environments that foster change in determinants

There are few studies of outcome evaluations of interventions in Western developed settings. The review identified only one study in Texas that examined the effect of a community based intervention on the use of child restraints in motorized transport [43]. The authors found that the intervention positively influenced safety behaviors such as the use of child restraints, drivers using seat belts and children riding in the back seat. Johnson has argued that while the study outcomes are likely the direct result of the intervention's efforts, any links to the 'safe community' designation are at best tenuous. He recommends that future studies should explore the interaction between safe community designation and injury prevention programs and define success not only by outcomes but also process dynamics such as reach, sustainability of efforts and pathways of change [55].

3.5. Smart Growth Planning

Smart Growth (or Smart Growth Planning) is a philosophy that strategically directs urban development activities in order to promote environmental sustainability, economic revitalization and sense of community. While there is a burgeoning body of research that links urban form, physical activity and obesity the evidence linking Smart Growth and improved health outcomes is still emerging [56,57]. Only one article was identified that sought to explicitly connect Smart Growth Planning with physical activity [44]. The authors did not find a statistically significant increase in moderate to vigorous physical activity among children in smart growth communities compared to control communities. These results may be explained by a number of study limitations including small sample size, measurement of physical activity on the weekend only and subjective reporting of physical context.

There are too few studies that explore the effect of Smart Growth Planning on health outcomes. Future studies are needed that employ more robust designs with larger sample sizes, fuller complement of health outcome measures, and adequate periods of follow up to assess whether there is a critical time period for impacting health outcomes. There is also the need for a public health component of Smart Growth Planning that would facilitate mapping of principles to established community health goals as part of project evaluations.

3.6. Other Healthy Community Approaches

There is a dearth of studies that met the inclusion criteria related to Healthy Cities, Child Friendly Cities, Livable Cities, Social Cities and Dementia Friendly Cities. A closer examination of the literature provided a number of plausible explanations for the gaps in knowledge about whether these approaches result in measureable improvements in the health of populations.

Some approaches are relatively new and or emerging hence more work is needed to bring conceptual clarity in order to define criteria for designation and facilitate evaluation of projects. This is the case for Dementia Friendly Cities where work has begun to define the features of the home and built environment that facilitate ease of navigation by persons with dementia who often have sensory and cognitive deficits [58–60]. The literature related to Social Cities is also very scant and further work to promote coherence and definition of the concept needs to be undertaken so that it becomes a discrete and measurable entity. Once consensus is achieved on established criteria and experience with implementation grows, evidence can more easily be generated on any associated benefits and outcomes on quality of life and wellbeing.

The concept of livability has received growing attention over time. While there is general consensus that it refers to desirable characteristics of the social, physical and economic infrastructures of cities and towns, a common definition has been elusive [61]. Consequently, "livable" communities reflect a confluence of healthy community approaches that find unique expression in individual cities. Although all members of the society are intended beneficiaries of efforts to create livable communities, the concept has often been viewed from the perspective of older persons who comprise a growing segment of the population and for whom independent living and aging in place are contingent on a supportive environment.

A search of the literature revealed several tools and checklists for assessing characteristics of communities. There were several narrative reports that described conceptual frameworks or achievements of initiatives such as the Partnership for Sustainable Communities Initiative (US) [62], and Livable Centers Initiative [63]; however, efforts to locate studies and evaluation reports that included quantifiable health outcomes were unsuccessful. This is surprising given that improvement in the quality of life is often an explicit objective of programs that address livability [64]. Studies are needed that explore the health benefits for communities willing to employ those strategies.

The complex nature of the approach also poses challenges for the assessment of impact on health outcomes. Both approaches that support the development of Healthy Cities and Child Friendly Cities are broad in scope and seek to impact health through distal upstream efforts. Additionally, both approaches emphasize the process of implementation and focus on the creation of supportive environments through the development of enabling multisectoral structures and community assets [65,66]. The emphasis on development of an inclusive collaborative process may also result in a relative neglect of measurement of health outcomes as milestones of success. These challenges may be addressed with the use of alternative evaluation approaches such as social return on investment [67], realist evaluation [68] and outcome mapping [69]. While they are distinctly different methodologies, they allow for broader conceptualization of the value of a program from the perspective of stakeholders and may better accommodate complexity while providing even more comprehensive answers about how programs work and in what settings. A common set of outcomes including self-rated health and percentage time spent in moderate to vigorous physical activity may be useful program impact indicators.

The gap in the literature with respect to evidence of the effectiveness of Healthy Cities has been recognized. There is still considerable international debate about evaluation needs and methods [70,71]. The current research emphasis remains on questions related to the process of implementation (what works and what does not, and why, in the implementation process of a complex intervention such as this) with the expectation, of course, that changes in the social determinants cascade will impact health and well-being of communities. Without a clear mandate and consensus on how the value of healthy communities should be judged, this is likely to hamper work in this area.

There are several limitations of the study that should be considered in the context of its results. The scope of the review is limited to studies pertaining to selected healthy community approaches. As a result of the focused examination, extrapolation of the results to other approaches is limited. Initiatives were not equally represented in US and Canadian jurisdictions with the latter contributing fewer studies. Despite efforts to search the grey literature, many of the programs were implemented by institutions or community organizations at the local level and may not have been published in the public domain. There were few studies that were identified and employed a rigorous design that would allow for strong causal inference. This meant that available studies were not well suited to explore research questions related to the program impact. While this does not imply that the studies do not contain valuable information, it highlights the need for more research that examines what works and under what circumstances.

4. Conclusions

The body of research to support the effectiveness of selected healthy community approaches on health outcomes is limited, mainly in terms of both the depth of the evidence base and the rigor of the studies. Despite the fact that it seems reasonable, based on underlying explanatory frameworks, to suggest that healthy community approaches should be effective, there is relatively little confirmation provided by the literature. In many instances, communities and institutions lack the enabling resources (expertise, time and finances) to conduct an evaluation or do not prioritize evaluation alongside program implementation. Without adequate provisions to collect baseline data, this compromises future efforts to determine program effectiveness. Consequently, the majority of studies employed a quasi-experimental or observational design with the attendant limitations that result from lack of random allocation or absence of a concurrent or well-delineated comparison group. There is also a notable absence of theory that guides studies related to most healthy community approaches that were examined. Other frequent flaws encountered included failure to control for potential confounding factors; reliance on subjective assessment of the outcomes to the exclusion of more objective measures that can be verified and duration of follow up that was inadequate to determine if any observed changes were sustained. In the case of Safe Routes to School programs and ALbD projects where the necessary support and priority is accorded to evaluation, more studies have been conducted.

A related issue that affects the availability of evidence of effectiveness is the differential emphasis on evaluation of the process of implementation over outcomes. Healthy community approaches depend on the establishment of multisectoral partnerships to achieve their goals. In many instances, benchmark criteria require demonstration of these collaborative processes for legitimacy. There is a need to promote more comprehensive approaches to evaluation that address structure, process and outcome components and better satisfy the information needs of all stakeholders.

Although there are inherent difficulties with attribution of observed outcomes to interventions with observational designs, there is weak evidence to support an association between selected healthy community approaches and achievement of positive health outcomes. The majority of included studies pertained to Safe Routes to School Programs and reported consistent positive association between students' active commute and program implementation. Safety benefits and changes in physical activity levels need to be confirmed with further studies. There is a paucity of studies about Active Living Communities, Age-Friendly Cities, Safe Communities and Smart Growth Planning. The evidence base needs to be strengthened by additional studies that are conceptualized to assess the effect of multifaceted interventions that may exert an influence synergistically or on specific health outcomes.

Several approaches including Healthy Cities/Communities, Child Friendly Cities, Dementia Friendly Cities and Social Cities have been relatively less studied in terms of health outcomes. The process of implementation has traditionally been emphasized in Healthy Cities and Child Friendly Cities given their focus on influencing policy to address broad social determinants. Research on these approaches is likely to be driven by practical considerations, relevance and utility in the specific city/community context. The latter two approaches (Dementia Friendly and Social Cities) require consensus and definition of uniform criteria to support design of interventions that can be evaluated.

Acknowledgments: The work was supported by the Public Health Agency of Canada (contract # 4500309324).

Author Contributions: The study was conceived and designed by BJ, NM and SJ. HW conducted the search, abstracted the data elements, and wrote the manuscript. All authors contributed to the interpretation of the findings and preparation of the manuscript.

Conflicts of Interest: The authors declare no conflict of interest.

Abbreviations

ASRTS	Active and Safe Routes to School;
ALbD	Active Living by Design;
CDC	Centers for Disease Control;
EPPHP	Effective Public Health Practice Project;
NTL	National Transportation Library;
SAFETEA-LU	Safe Accountable Flexible Efficient Transportation Equity Act: A Legacy for Users;
STP	School Travel Planning;
SRTS	Safe Routes to School;
UNICEF	United Nations Children Fund;
WHO	World Health Organization;
WSB	Walking School Bus.

Appendix: Search Strategy for Safe Routes to School

Medline OVID SP (2000–2014)

(i) Walking/
(i) Bicycling/
(i) Transportation/
(i) 1 or 2 or 3
(i) Safety/
(i) Schools/
(i) Child/
(i) 4 and 5 and 6 and 7

SCOPUS (Limits to English, 2000–2014)

(i) Safe Routes to School

References and Notes

1. Commission on Social Determinants of Health (CSDH). *Closing the Gap in a Generation: Health Equity through Action on the Social Determinants of Health. Final Report of the Commission on Social Determinants of Health.* Geneva: World Health Organization, 2008. Available online: http://www.who.int/social_determinants/thecommission/finalreport/en/ (accessed on 10 October 2014).

2. Timothy Evans, Margaret Whitehead, Finn Diderichsen, Abbas Bhuiya and Meg Wirth. *Challenging Inequities in Health Care: From Ethics to Action*. New York: Oxford University Press, 2001; pp. 309–22.
3. Trevor Hancock. Act Locally: Community-based population health promotion. Available online: http://www.parl.gc.ca/Content/SEN/Committee/402/popu/rep/appendixBjun09-e.pdf (accessed on 7 August 2015).
4. National Research Council and Institute of Medicine. *U.S. Health in International Perspective: Shorter Lives, Poorer Health. Panel on Understanding Cross-National Health Differences among High-Income Countries*. Edited by Steven H. Woolf and Aron Laudan. Washington: The National Academies Press, 2013.
5. Tyler Norris, and Mary Pittman. " The healthy communities movement and the coalition for healthier cities and communities." *Public Health Reports* 115 (2000): 118.
6. UNICEF Innocenti Research Centre. Building Child Friendly Cities: A framework for action. Available online: http://childfriendlycities.org/wp_content/uploads/2013/04/pdf/BuildingCFC_AFrameworkforaction_en.pdf (accessed on 9 September 2015).
7. Smart Growth Online. What is smart growth? Available online: http://www.smartgrowth.org/what-is-smart-growth/ (accessed on 9 September 2015).
8. National Center for Safe Routes to School. Available online: http://saferoutesinfo.org/about-us/history-srts (accessed on 9 September 2015).
9. WHO Collaborating Centre on Community Safety Promotion. Available online: http://isccc.global/how-to-become-an-international-safe-community (accessed on 25 December 2015).
10. Active Living Research. Available online: http://activelivingresearch.org/active-living-topics (accessed on 9 September 2015).
11. Elizabeth E. Fischer. " Building livable communities for the 21st century." *Public Roads* 63 (2000): 30–34.
12. Cardus. About the Social Cities Research Program. Available online: http://www.cardus.ca/research/socialcities/ (accessed on 9 September 2015).
13. World Health Organization. Global Age Friendly Cities: A Guide. Available online: http://apps.who.int/iris/bitstream/10665/43755/1/9/8921 (accessed on 9 September 2015).
14. Alzheimer's Society. Dementia Friendly Communities. Available online: http://www.alzheimers.org.uk/site/scripts/documents_info.php?documentID=1843 (accessed on 10 September 2015).
15. Noreen C. McDonald, Pamela H. Barth, and Ruth L. Steiner. " Assessing the Distribution of Safe Routes to School Program Funds, 2005–2012." *American Journal of Preventive Medicine* 45 (2013): 401–6.
16. Angie L. Cradock, Billy Fields, Jessica L. Barrett, and Steven Melly. " Program practices and demographic factors associated with federal funding for the Safe Routes to School program in the United States." *Health & Place* 18 (2012): 16–23.

17. Philip Bors, Mark Dessauer, Rich Bell, Risa Wilkerson, Joanne Lee, and Sarah L. Strunk. " The Active Living by Design national program: Community initiatives and lessons learned." *American Journal of Preventive Medicine* 37 (2009): S313–21.
18. Lynn Weigand. A review of literature: The effectiveness of Safe Routes to School and other programs to promote active transportation to school. Available online: https://www.pdx.edu/ibpi/ sites/www.pdx.edu.ibpi/files/Safe%20Routes%20White%20Paper.pdf (accessed on 25 August 2015).
19. Anneliese Spinks, Cathy Turner, Jim Nixon, and Roderick J. McClure. " The WHO Safe Communities model for the prevention of injury in whole populations." *Cochrane Database of Systematic Reviews* 3 (2009): CD004445.
20. Effective Public Health Practice Project. "Quality Assessment Tool for Quantitative Studies." Available online: http://www.ephpp.ca/Tools.html (accessed on 7 August 2015).
21. Jason A. Mendoza, David D. Levinger, and Brian D. Johnston. " Pilot evaluation of a walking school bus program in a low-income, urban community." *BMC Public Health* 9 (2009): 122.
22. Jason A. Mendoza, Kathy Watson, Tom Baranowski, Theresa A. Nicklas, Doris K. Uscanga, and Marcus J. Hanfling. " The walking school bus and children's physical activity: A pilot cluster randomized controlled trial." *Pediatrics* 128 (2011): e537–44.
23. Marlon G. Boarnet, Craig L. Anderson, Kristen Day, Tracy McMillan, and Mariela Alfonzo. " Evaluation of the California Safe Routes to School legislation: Urban form changes and children's active transportation to school." *American Journal of Preventive Medicine* 28 (2005): 134–40.
24. Jill F. Cooper and Tracy E. McMillan. "Safe Routes to School Local School Project: A health evaluation at 10 low income schools." Available online: http://saferoutespartnership.org/ sites/ default/files/pdf/Health_Evaluation_Feb_2010.pdf (accessed on 8 August 2015).
25. Ron Buliung, Guy Faulkner, Theresa Beesley, and Jacky Kennedy. " School travel planning: Mobilizing school and community resources to encourage active school transportation." *Journal of School Health* 81 (2011): 704–12.
26. George Mammen, Michelle R. Stone, Guy Faulkner, Subha Ramanathan, Ron Buliung, Catherine O'Brien, and Jacky Kennedy. " Active school travel: An evaluation of the Canadian school travel planning intervention." *Preventive Medicine* 60 (2014): 55–59.
27. Susan Henderson, Robin Tanner, Norma Klanderman, Abby Mattera, Lindsey Martin Webb, and John Steward. " Safe Routes to School: A public health practice success story—Atlanta, 2008–2010." *Journal of Physical Activity and Health* 10 (2013): 141–42.
28. Noreen C. McDonald, Yizhao Yang, Steve M. Abbott, and Allison N. Bullock. " Impact of the Safe Routes to School program on walking and biking: Eugene, Oregon study." *Transport Policy* 29 (2013): 243–48.

29. Noreen C. McDonald, Ruth L. Steiner, Chanam Lee, Tori Rhoulac Smith, Xuemei Zhu, and Yizhao Yang. "Impact of the safe routes to school program on walking and bicycling." *Journal of the American Planning Association* 80 (2014): 153–67.
30. Anne Vernez Moudon, and Orion Stewart. "Moving forward: Safe Routes to School progress in five states." Available online: http://www.wsdot.wa.gov/research/reports/fullreports/743.3.pdf (accessed on 8 August 2015).
31. Catherine E. Staunton, Deb Hubsmith, and Wendi Kallins. "Promoting safe walking and biking to school: The Marin County success story." *American Journal of Public Health* 93 (2003): 1431–34.
32. Aaron Buckley, Michael B. Lowry, Helen Brown, and Benjamin Barton. "Evaluating safe routes to school events that designate days for walking and bicycling." *Transport Policy* 30 (2013): 294–300.
33. Brian D. Johnston, Jason Mendoza, Sarah Rafton, Denise Gonzalez-Walker, and David Levinger. "Promoting physical activity and reducing child pedestrian risk: Early evaluation of a walking school bus program in central Seattle." *Journal of Trauma and Acute Care Surgery* 60 (2006): 1388–89.
34. Stephen P. Sayers, Joseph W. LeMaster, Ian M. Thomas, Gregory F. Petroski, and Bin Ge. "A Walking School Bus program: Impact on physical activity in elementary school children in Columbia, Missouri." *American Journal of Preventive Medicine* 43 (2012): S384–89.
35. Charles DiMaggio, and Guohua Li. "Effectiveness of a safe routes to school program in preventing school-aged pedestrian injury." *Pediatrics* 131 (2013): 290–96.
36. Richard D. Blomberg, Arlene M. Cleven, F. Dennis Thomas III, and Raymond C. Peck. *Evaluation of the Safety Benefits of Legacy Safe Routes to School Programs*. Washington: National Highway Traffic Safety Administration, 2008. Available online: http://www.nhtsa.gov/DOT/NHTSA/Communication%20.../tt368.pdf (accessed on 8 August 2015).
37. Marla R. Orenstein, Nicolas Gutierrez, Thomas M. Rice, Jill F. Cooper, and David R. Ragland. *Safe Routes to School Safety and Mobility Analysis*. Berkley: UC Berkley Traffic Safety Center, 2007. Available online: http://www.dot.ca.gov/hq/LocalPrograms/saferoutes/documents/SR2S+Final_Report_to_the_Legislature.pdf (accessed on 9 August 2015).
38. David R. Ragland, Swati Pande, John Bigham, and Jill F. Cooper. "Ten years later: Examining the long term impact of the California Safe Routes to School Program." Paper presented at the Transportation Research Board 93rd Annual Meeting, Washington, DC, USA, 12–16 January 2014. Available online: http://doc.trb.org/prp/14-4226.pdf (accessed on 25 December 2015).
39. Jason A. Mendoza, Kathy Watson, Tzu-An Chen, Tom Baranowski, Theresa A. Nicklas, Doris K. Uscanga, and Marcus J. Hanfling. "Impact of a pilot walking school bus intervention on children's pedestrian safety behaviors: A pilot study." *Health & Place* 18 (2012): 24–30.

40. Virginia R. Chomitz, Julia C. McDonald, Denise B. Aske, Lisa N. Arsenault, Nicole A. Rioles, Lisa B. Brukilacchio, Karen A. Hacker, and Howard J. Cabral. " Evaluation results from an active living intervention in Somerville, Massachusetts." *American Journal of Preventive Medicine* 43 (2012): S367–78.
41. David S. TenBrink, Randall McMunn, and Sarah Panken. " Project U-Turn: Increasing active transportation in Jackson, Michigan." *American Journal of Preventive Medicine* 37 (2009): S329–35.
42. Stephen P. Sayers, Joseph W. LeMaster, Ian M. Thomas, Gregory F. Petroski, and Bin Ge. " Bike, Walk, and Wheel: A way of life in Columbia, Missouri, revisited." *American Journal of Preventive Medicine* 43 (2012): S379–83.
43. Gregory R. Istre, Martha Stowe, Mary A. McCoy, Billy J. Moore, Dan Culica, Katie N. Womack, and Ron J. Anderson. " A controlled evaluation of the WHO Safe Communities model approach to injury prevention: Increasing child restraint use in motor vehicles." *Injury Prevention* 17 (2011): 3–8.
44. Genevieve F. Dunton, Stephen S. Intille, Jennifer Wolch, and Mary Ann Pentz. " Investigating the impact of a smart growth community on the contexts of children's physical activity using Ecological Momentary Assessment." *Health & Place* 18 (2012): 76–84.
45. Amanda J. Lehning, Richard J. Smith, and Ruth E. Dunkle. " Age-Friendly Environments and Self-Rated Health: An Exploration of Detroit Elders." *Research on Aging* 36 (2012): 72–94.
46. Verena H. Menec, and Scott Nowicki. " Examining the relationship between communities' 'age-friendliness' and life satisfaction and self-perceived health in rural Manitoba, Canada." *Rural and Remote Health* 14 (2014): 1–14. Available online: http://www.rrh.org.au/articles/subviewnew.asp?ArticleID=2594 (accessed on 25 December 2015).
47. Kim L. Bercovitz, and Harvey A Skinner. " Active Living—Just a passing fad? " *Canadain Journal of Public Health* 87 (1996): 275–79.
48. Elaine Gallagher, and Angie Mallhi. " Age-Friendly British Columbia. Lessons learned from October 1, 2007–September 30, 2010." Available online: http://www2.gov.bc.ca/assets/gov/ people/seniors/about-seniorsbc/afbc/afbc_ evaluation_ report.pdf (accessed on 25 December 2015).
49. Neil Steffler, and Lisa Kaldeway. "City of Kawartha Lakes Age-Friendly Project Assessment: Report to the Community, 2011." Available online: http://www.hkpr.on.ca/Portals/0/ PDF%20Files%20-%20CDIP/AFReport-web.pdf (accessed on 10 October 2014).
50. Verena H. Menec, Sheila Novek, Dawn Veselyuk, and Jennifer McArthur. " Lessons learned from a Canadian province-wide age-friendly initiative: The Age-Friendly Manitoba Initiative." *Journal of Aging & Social Policy* 26 (2014): 33–51.

51. Mary Wiley. "Niagara Age-Friendly Community Initiative Year 1 2010–2011. Evaluation Report." Available online: https://notl.civicweb.net/document/3543/Niagara%20Age-Friendly%20Summary%20Report.pdf?handle=0A6A4D09624A46BF808D78BEB6BFA16F (accessed on 25 December 2015).
52. WHO Centre for Health Development. "2nd WHO Consultation on Developing Indicators for Age-Friendly Cities." 8 September 2013. Available online: http://www.seniorscouncil.net/uploads/files/AFC_Mtg-2_Report_SEP2013_Quebec.pdf (accessed on 14 August 2015).
53. Parachute. Available online: http://www.parachutecanada.org/safecommunities (accessed on 6 September 2015).
54. Nilsen Per. " What makes community based injury injury prevention work? In search of evidence of effectiveness." *Injury Prevention* 10 (2004): 268–274.
55. Brian D. Johnston. " Injury prevention in safe communities." *Injury Prevention* 17 (2011): 1–2.
56. Casey P. Durand, Mohammad Andalib, Genevieve F. Dunton, Jennifer Wolch, and Mary Ann Pentz. " A systematic review of built environment factors related to physical activity and obesity risk: Implications for smart growth urban planning." *Obesity Reviews* 12 (2011): e173–82.
57. Nazeem Muhajarine. " Canadian Evidence on Built Environment and Health." *Canadian Journal of Public Health* 103 (2012): S3–72.
58. Lynne Mitchell, Elizabeth Burton, and Shibu Raman. " Dementia-friendly cities: Intelligible neighbourhoods for life." *Journal of Urban Design* 9 (2004): 89–101.
59. Lynne Mitchell. Breaking New Ground. "The Quest for Dementia-Friendly Communities." 2012. Available online: www.housinglin.org.uk (accessed on 14 September 2015).
60. Jason Su. " Built for Dementia: Urban Design analysis for Dementia-Friendly Communities." Master Thesis, San Jose State University, San Jose, CA, USA, 1 April 2013. Available online: http://scholarworks.sjsu.edu/cgi/viewcontent.cgi?article=1317&context=etd_projects (accessed on 25 December 2015).
61. Matthias Ruth, and Rachel S. Franklin. " Livability for all? Conceptual limits and practical limitations." *Applied Geography* 49 (2014): 18–23.
62. Partnership for Sustainable Communities. Available online: https://www.sustainablecommunities.gov/mission/livability-principles (accessed on 6 September 2015).
63. Atlanta Regional Commission. "Livable Centers Initiative (LCI) Implementation Report." 2013. Available online: http://www.atlantaregional.com/land-use/livable-centers-initiative (accessed on 10 August 2015).
64. Partners for Livable Communities. Available online: http://livable.org (accessed on 6 September 2015).
65. Silvie Schulze, and Francesca Moneti. " The Child Friendly Cities Initiative." *Municipal Engineer* 160 (2007): 77–81.

66. World Health Organization. "Healthy Settings." 2014. Available online: http://www.who.int/ healthy_settings/types/cities/en (accessed on 6 September 2015).
67. Malin Arvidson, Fergus Lyon, Stephen McKay, and Domenico Moro. "The ambitions and challenges of SROI." *Third Sector Research Centre*, 2010. Available online: https://eprints.mdx.ac.uk/7104/1/The_ambitions_and_challenges_of_SROI.pdf (accessed on 6 September 2015).
68. Ray Pawson, and Nick Tilley. *Realistic Evaluation*. London: Sage, 1997.
69. Sarah Earl, Fred Carden, and Terry Smutylo. *Outcome Mapping. Building Learning and Reflection into Development Programs*. Ottawa: International Development Research Centre, 2001. Available online: http://www.outcomemapping.ca/download.php?file=/resource/files/OM_English_final.pdf (accessed on 25 December 2015).
70. Evelyne De Leeuw, and Thomas Skovgaard. " Utility-driven evidence for healthy cities: Problems with evidence generation and application." *Social Science & Medicine* 61 (2005): 1331–41.
71. Evelyne De Leeuw. "Evaluating WHO Healthy Cities in Europe: Issues and perspectives." *Journal of Urban Health* 90 (2013): 14–22.

MDPI AG

St. Alban-Anlage 66

4052 Basel, Switzerland

Tel. +41 61 683 77 34

Fax +41 61 302 89 18

http://www.mdpi.com

Social Sciences Editorial Office

E-mail: socsci@mdpi.com

http://www.mdpi.com/journal/socsci

www.ingramcontent.com/pod-product-compliance
Lightning Source LLC
LaVergne TN
LVHW070416100526
838202LV00014B/1468